Human Embryology
The Ultimate USMLE
Step 1
Review

Human Embryology

The Ultimate USMLE Step 1 Review

Philip R. Brauer, Ph.D.
Associate Professor
Department of Biomedical Sciences
Creighton University School of Medicine
Omaha, Nebraska

HANLEY & BELFUS
An Imprint of Elsevier

HANLEY & BELFUS, INC.
An Imprint of Elsevier

The Curtis Center
Independence Square West
Philadelphia, Pennsylvania 19106

Note to the reader: Although the techniques, ideas, and information in this book have been carefully reviewed for correctness, neither the author nor the publisher can accept any legal responsibility for any errors or omissions that may be made. Neither the author nor the publisher makes any guarantee, expressed or implied, with respect to the material contained herein.

Library of Congress Control Number: 2002117749

HUMAN EMBRYOLOGY: THE ULTIMATE USMLE STEP I REVIEW   ISBN 1-56053-561-X

Printed in Canada

Last digit is the print number: 9   8   7   6   5   4   3   2   1

Contents

Preface

Over the past several decades, medical knowledge has grown by leaps and bounds. Yet, at most institutions the medical school curriculum is still taught in 4 years. For students, not only is it difficult to assimilate the essential background knowledge within this time frame, but it is even more difficult to retain it. However, students are particularly adept at recalling a lot of information with only a cursory glance over synopses, illustrations, and outlines. The goal of this book is to provide a tool enabling students to recall many of the details regarding human development and congenital diseases that they may have been exposed to in several courses or over a period of several years.

Congenital anomalies are the leading cause of infant death. Approximately 2%–3% of all newborns exhibit at least 1 recognizable congenital anomaly, and many pathologies seen in adults are due to congenital anomalies. Recognizing these facts, students, particularly those preparing for licensing exams, want a concise and inclusive review of human embryology. For those preparing for licensing exams, this book should provide a quick and efficient review of human embryology. For others, this book may serve as a brief introduction to the subject. Each chapter consists of a single page of diagrams coupled with a single page of text, which includes a very brief overview of each chapter. This book is divided into 3 parts. After each part, a series of practice questions follow to test the reader's recollection and understanding of basic principles related to human embryology.

I hope that all readers find this book useful, as that is my intent.

Philip R. Brauer

Dedication

To Tracy, for without her love and support I could not have written this book. And to Bobo and April, who sacrificed their playtime to make this book possible. I am one lucky dog.

Acknowledgments

I wish to thank my colleagues at Creighton University for inspiring me to be a better teacher and for sharing their teaching experiences with me. I would also like to thank my past mentors, Drs. Don A. Hay, Roger R. Markwald, and John M. Keller, who showed me that a person can be an excellent and dedicated teacher and also make contributions toward expanding scientific knowledge.

Abbreviations

ACTH	adrenocorticotropin		LH	luteinizing hormone
AV	atrioventricular (node)		MIS	müllerian-inhibiting substance
cm	centimeter		mg	milligrams
CSF	cerebrospinal fluid		mL	milliliter
ES	embryonic stem (cells)		mm	millimeter
FSH	follicle-stimulating hormone		MRI	magnetic resonance imaging
GI	gastrointestinal		NTD	neural tube defect
gm	gram		PCR	polymerase chain reaction
GnRH	gonadotropin-releasing hormone		RBC	red blood cell
hCG	human choriogonadotropin		SA	sinoatrial (node)
HIV	human immunodeficiency virus		TDF	testis-determining factor
IUGR	intrauterine growth restriction		VSD	ventricular septal defect

PART I

1 Mitosis and Meiosis

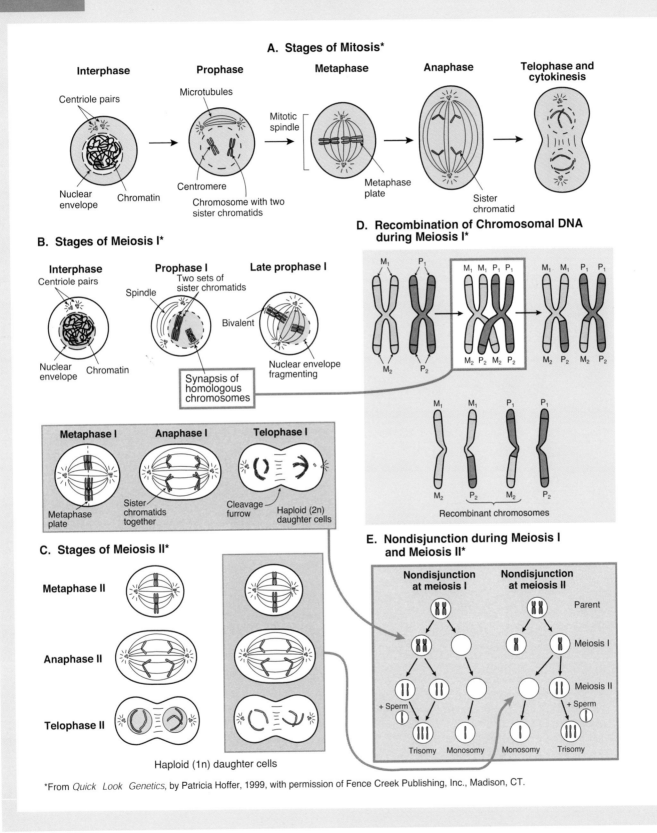

A. Stages of Mitosis*

Interphase — Centriole pairs, Nuclear envelope, Chromatin

Prophase — Microtubules, Centromere, Chromosome with two sister chromatids

Metaphase — Mitotic spindle, Metaphase plate

Anaphase — Sister chromatid

Telophase and cytokinesis

B. Stages of Meiosis I*

Interphase — Centriole pairs, Nuclear envelope, Chromatin

Prophase I — Spindle, Two sets of sister chromatids

Late prophase I — Bivalent, Nuclear envelope fragmenting

Synapsis of homologous chromosomes

Metaphase I — Metaphase plate

Anaphase I — Sister chromatids together

Telophase I — Cleavage furrow, Haploid (2n) daughter cells

C. Stages of Meiosis II*

Metaphase II

Anaphase II

Telophase II

Haploid (1n) daughter cells

D. Recombination of Chromosomal DNA during Meiosis I*

M_1 P_1 → M_1 M_1 P_1 P_1 → M_1 M_1 P_1 P_1

M_2 P_2 M_2 P_2 M_2 P_2 M_2 P_2 M_2 P_2

M_1 M_1 P_1 P_1

M_2 P_2 M_2 P_2

Recombinant chromosomes

E. Nondisjunction during Meiosis I and Meiosis II*

Nondisjunction at meiosis I | **Nondisjunction at meiosis II**

Parent

Meiosis I

Meiosis II

+ Sperm

Trisomy — Monosomy — Monosomy — Trisomy

+ Sperm

*From *Quick Look Genetics*, by Patricia Hoffer, 1999, with permission of Fence Creek Publishing, Inc., Madison, CT.

OVERVIEW

The human karyotype consists of 46 strands of DNA arranged as 23 pairs (diploid), one strand of paternal origin and the other of maternal origin (2n). Before mitosis, each strand is replicated during the S-phase. During early mitosis, these strands condense into chromosomes. The chromosomes then separate so that each daughter cell is an exact genetic replica of the parent. Meiosis produces germ cells that contain either the paternal or the maternal chromosome of a chromosome pair (haploid) and only a single DNA copy (1n). Meiosis involves 2 cycles of cell division. In meiosis I, homologous paternal and maternal chromosomes pair up and align at the metaphase plate, and the paternal or maternal copy of each pair segregates into different daughter cells (now haploid and 2n). Meiosis II resembles mitosis but commences without an intervening S-phase. After meiosis II is complete, the germ cells are still haploid but 1n. Many chromosomal anomalies result from abnormal meiosis I or II, and many are lethal.

Human Karyotype

The human karyotype consists of 46 strands or 23 pairs of DNA strands called *chromatin*. There are 22 pairs of autosomal chromatin and 1 pair of sex chromatin. One member of each pair is of maternal origin and the other is of paternal origin, each coding the same type of information. These chromatin pairs are often referred to as *homologous pairs,* but during interphase they are usually distributed separately within the nucleus. Cells containing a paired configuration of chromatin are called *diploid cells,* and before the S-phase of the cell cycle there is a single copy of the paternal and maternal chromatin (2n for each homologous pair). When the S-phase is complete, the paternal and maternal chromatin strands have been duplicated, and the original and replica strands are held together by a *centromere*. At this point, there are 4 strands of DNA for each homologous pair (4n). During mitosis, these duplicated chromatin strands condense into chromosomes, with each individual DNA strand being referred to as a *chromatid.*

Mitosis

Mitosis is the process of cell division whereby the daughter cells are an exact genetic replica of each other and the parent (**Part A**). This is accomplished by karyokinesis (chromosomal duplication and separation) and cytokinesis (splitting of the cytoplasm). Each daughter cell receives 1 copy of each duplicated chromatin strand. The steps of karyokinesis are:

1. Replication of DNA during the S-phase of the cell cycle
2. Condensing of the duplicated DNA strands into chromosomes that are held together by a centromere (prophase)
3. Chromosomal attachment to the mitotic spindle and alignment along the midline (metaphase)
4. Separation of the chromatids at the centromere (anaphase)
5. Nuclear envelope formation, decondensation of the chromatid, and completion of cytokinesis (telophase)

Meiosis

Mitosis, while well suited for replacing cells or replicating single-cell organisms, does not lend itself well to the reproduction of entire multicellular organisms. More complicated organisms replicate through sexual reproduction. Here, the genomes of 2 separate individuals are mixed to produce offspring that are genetically different from their siblings and from both parents.

The purpose of meiosis is to generate gametes that are haploid and 1n and provide genetic variability through the process of random genetic recombination and crossover. Meiosis is accomplished through 2 separate and consecutive cell divisions referred to as *meiosis I* and *meiosis II* (**Parts B** and **C**). Meiosis begins with the replication of DNA and condensation into chromosomes. However, during prophase I of meiosis I, the paternal and maternal chromosomes of each pair align

with one another point to point in a process called *synapsis*. During this stage, genetic material is exchanged between paternal and maternal homologous segments through a process called *crossover* (discussed below). During metaphase I, homologous pairs become connected to one another, attach to the mitotic spindle, and align along the equatorial plate. At this point, the paternal chromosome of a pair will be facing one pole and the maternal chromosome facing the other (facing direction is random for each homologous pair). During anaphase I, the paternal and maternal chromosomes migrate to opposite poles, but the centromere holding the duplicated strands does not split during meiosis I. After telophase I, each daughter cell then contains either the maternal or the paternal representative of each homologous pair but not both (haploid). However, each daughter cell contains DNA replicas of the paternal or maternal chromatin (2n). Meiosis II then proceeds much like mitosis, with the exception that there is no intervening DNA synthesis. Therefore, after meiosis II, each daughter cell (now a germ cell) is still haploid but 1n.

Possible Gamete Types

In humans, the number of genetically different gametes that is mathematically possible based on 23 chromosome pairs is 2^{23} or 8.4×10^6. Actually, the number of variants produced is much higher because of a second type of reassortment called *chromosomal crossover*. Chromosomal crossover takes place during meiosis I (**Part D**). During synapsis, homologous segments are exchanged between the maternal and paternal chromosomes. Crossover involves breaking the DNA double helix in the maternal chromosome and in the exact homologous region of the paternal chromosome, followed by an exchange of the DNA fragments. The maternal and paternal homologues are physically connected to each other at these points and produce X-like morphological structures between the chromosome pairs called *chiasmata*. Chiasmata are an important part of chromosomal segregation, as they hold the maternal and paternal homologues together on the spindle during metaphase I. Crossover permits an almost infinite amount of genetic diversity.

Clinical Aspects

Occasionally, abnormal meiotic divisions occur whereby both members of a chromosome pair move into the same daughter cell. This is referred to as *nondisjunction* (**Part E**). If the resulting germ cells combine with a normal germ-cell counterpart during fertilization, the karyotype of the offspring would be either trisomy or monosomy for that particular chromosome type. Nondisjunction can occur in both autosomes and sex chromosomes, leading to many congenital anomalies and spontaneous abortion. Abnormal crossover events, deletions, and duplications of chromosomes also can occur, leading to congenital defects, some of which are discussed in Chapter 46.

2 Female Gametogenesis

A. Origin of Primordial Germ Cells

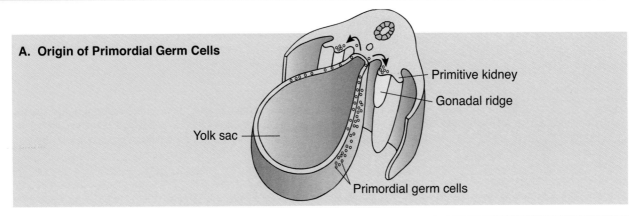

Primitive kidney

Gonadal ridge

Yolk sac

Primordial germ cells

B. Oogenesis in a 2-Chromosome (1-Pair) Organism

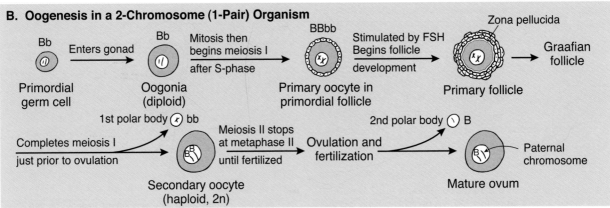

Bb

Enters gonad

Bb

Mitosis then begins meiosis I after S-phase

BBbb

Stimulated by FSH Begins follicle development

Zona pellucida

Graafian follicle

Primordial germ cell

Oogonia (diploid)

Primary oocyte in primordial follicle

Primary follicle

1st polar body bb

Completes meiosis I just prior to ovulation

Meiosis II stops at metaphase II until fertilized

Ovulation and fertilization

2nd polar body B

Paternal chromosome

Secondary oocyte (haploid, 2n)

Mature ovum

C. Follicle Development

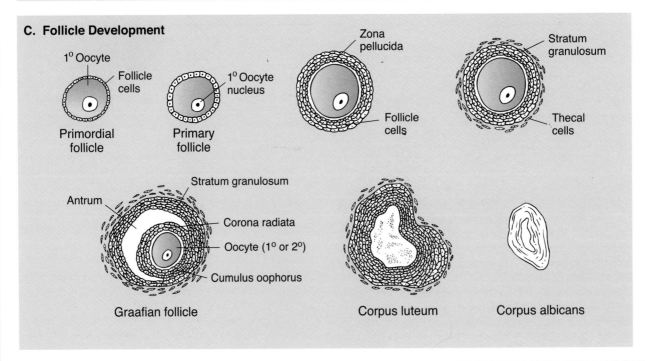

1^0 Oocyte

Follicle cells

Primordial follicle

1^0 Oocyte nucleus

Primary follicle

Zona pellucida

Follicle cells

Stratum granulosum

Thecal cells

Antrum

Stratum granulosum

Corona radiata

Oocyte (1^0 or 2^0)

Cumulus oophorus

Graafian follicle

Corpus luteum

Corpus albicans

OVERVIEW

Primordial germ cells in embryos with an XX karyotype differentiate into oogonia, divide, become surrounded by follicle cells in the developing ovary, and begin meiosis early in the fetal period. However, gametogenesis stops in meiosis I, and the oocyte within the follicle remains this way until puberty. Then every month until menopause, follicle-stimulating hormone (FSH) stimulates a few oocytes to continue meiosis, and the follicle cells begin secreting estrogen. Usually, only 1 oocyte is ovulated (the ovum). After ovulation, the remaining follicle cells transform into a temporary endocrine organ (the corpus luteum) that produces the progesterone and estrogen needed to ready the uterus for implantation. In the absence of fertilization, the corpus luteum degenerates in about 2 weeks, progesterone and estrogen levels drop, and menstruation begins. With pregnancy, the developing zygote releases hormones that maintain the corpus luteum until the placenta is capable of sustaining the pregnancy alone.

Primordial Germ Cells

Primordial germ cells are the ancestors of mature germ cells. Initially found during weeks 4–6 within the mesoderm of the yolk sac wall, primordial germ cells migrate through the yolk sac wall and mesentery and enter the genital ridge in the developing thoracic body wall (**Part A**). Once there, they proliferate and stimulate the surrounding cells to form sex cords. Sex cords eventually give rise to ovarian follicle cells (female) or Sertoli cells (male) (see Chapters 18 and 19). In females, primordial germ cells differentiate into oogonia and begin gametogenesis during the embryogenesis, whereas in males primordial germ cells do not differentiate into spermatogonia until puberty.

The Oogonia and Oocyte

The *oocyte* is the female gamete, and *oogenesis* is the process of oocyte development. In females, primordial germ cells proliferate and differentiate to generate several million oogonia. Oogonia then become surrounded by a layer of flattened follicular cells and differentiate into primary oocytes (**Parts B** and **C**). Primary oocytes start their first meiotic division during the embryonic and fetal period but are arrested in prophase I of meiosis. They remain in this state until stimulated to continue meiosis during the menstrual cycle. Many of these primary oocytes degenerate so that only about 40,000 remain by puberty. Of these, only a small number will be ovulated during the woman's entire lifetime.

Follicle Development

At the onset of puberty and every month until menopause, 5–15 primordial follicles, each containing a primary oocyte surrounded by follicular cells, are stimulated to begin development (**Part C**). Follicle cells proliferate, become multilayered, and together with the oocyte produce a thick protein membrane known as the *zona pellucida* separating the cells and the oocyte. Follicle cells become organized as a layer referred to as the *stratum granulosa* and begin producing estrogen. As the follicle enlarges, adjacent stromal cells become recruited into the follicle (thecal cells). As the follicle continues to increase in size, intercellular fluid accumulates, and fluid-filled spaces form between the granulosa cells and coalesce to form the follicular antrum. The antrum eventually enlarges to the point where the oocyte and surrounding granulosa cells become eccentrically placed. The hillock of granulosa cells is called the *cumulus oophorus,* and the layer of cells covering the oocyte is the *corona radiata*. At this point, the follicle is referred to as a *graafian follicle,* the last stage of follicle development before ovulation. Just before ovulation, the oocyte completes meiosis I to form a secondary oocyte that is now haploid. Division of the cytoplasm between the daughter cell is unequal; one oocyte gets almost all of the cytoplasm while the other oocyte gets very little. The small oocyte is referred to as a *polar body* and will eventually degenerate. The secondary oocyte begins meiosis II but becomes arrested in metaphase II and remains so until it is fertilized.

Ovulation

Ovulation occurs when the levels of FSH and luteinizing hormone (LH) peak during the menstrual cycle. In response to FSH and LH, the cumulus oophorus cells loosen, and the oocyte with the corona radiata detaches from the follicular wall. At the same time, follicular fluid increases, proteolytic enzymes begin to weaken the ovarian wall, and there is a concomitant decrease in blood flow to the tissue between the follicle and outer ovarian surface. These events lead to rupture of the ovarian wall and release of the ovum. Meanwhile, the oviduct becomes closely opposed to the ovarian surface, and beating cilia of the oviduct help sweep the ovum into the oviduct. This unfertilized ovum is viable for about 24 hours. If fertilization fails, the oocyte degenerates as it passes through the oviduct. Usually only 1 follicle is ovulated but occasionally more than 1 can be released, and if both are fertilized, the result is fraternal twins. Ovulation also can be induced by administration of gonadotropins or drugs like clomiphene citrate. These hormones and drugs stimulate the maturation of follicles and can lead to ovulation of multiple ova. With respect to the sex chromosome found in an ovum, normally only 1 kind of gamete can be generated, one with an X-sex chromosome.

Corpus Luteum

After release of the ovum, the remaining granulosa and thecal cells differentiate and form the *corpus luteum,* a temporary endocrine organ that synthesizes and secretes the progesterone and estrogen needed to prepare the endometrium of the uterus for implantation (**Part C**). If pregnancy does not occur, the corpus luteum atrophies in about 12–14 days and becomes the *corpus luteum of menstruation.* If fertilization and implantation begin, human choriogonadotropin (hCG) hormone synthesized by the developing embryo (primarily the syncytiotrophoblasts) maintains the corpus luteum until the placenta takes over its function. This is referred to as the *corpus luteum of pregnancy* and it will occupy most of the ovarian space. When the corpus luteum atrophies, connective tissue replaces the luteal cells, forming a scarlike structure in the ovary referred to as a *corpus albicans*. Follicles that never reach maturity and degenerate during fetal and early postnatal life or during the menstrual cycles are resorbed, autolyzed, and replaced with connective tissue. These follicles are referred to as *atretic follicles*.

Clinical Aspects

The likelihood of generating oocytes with chromosomal anomalies increases with age. In women approaching menopause, oocytes have been in an arrested state for 40–50 years before continuing with meiosis. This may be responsible, in part, for the increased frequency of nondisjunction of chromosomes in gametes observed with age.

3 The Menstrual Cycle

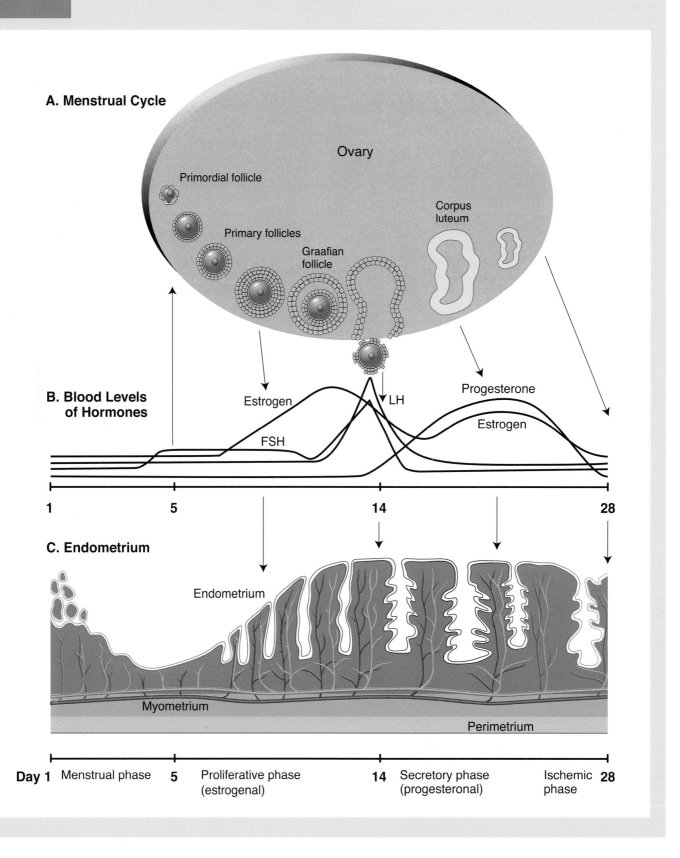

A. Menstrual Cycle

Ovary

Primordial follicle

Primary follicles

Graafian follicle

Corpus luteum

B. Blood Levels of Hormones

Estrogen

FSH

LH

Progesterone

Estrogen

1   5   14   28

C. Endometrium

Endometrium

Myometrium

Perimetrium

Day 1 Menstrual phase **5** Proliferative phase (estrogenal) **14** Secretory phase (progesteronal) Ischemic phase **28**

OVERVIEW

Major hormones of the menstrual cycle include two pituitary hormones, FSH and LH, and two gonadal hormones, estrogen and progesterone. FSH is responsible for initiating follicle development, stimulating estrogen synthesis and secretion by follicle cells, and together with LH, initiates ovulation. Regrowth of the endometrial mucosa after menstruation depends on estrogen. After ovulation, LH transforms the remaining follicle cells into the corpus luteum, which secretes progesterone and estrogen needed for preparing the endometrium for implantation. The reparative, proliferative, secretory, ischemic, and menstrual changes in the endometrium during the menstrual cycle are driven by gonadal hormones released by the cyclic development and degeneration of ovarian follicles.

Major Hormones Related to Menstrual Cycle

FSH and LH are both produced in the anterior pituitary in response to gonadotropin-releasing hormone (GnRH) released by the hypothalamus. Their primary target is the ovary. FSH is required for the initiation of follicular development during each menstrual cycle. In response to FSH, follicular cells synthesize and secrete estrogen (**Part A** and **B**). LH is involved in the final maturation of the follicle and after ovulation transforms the remaining follicle and thecal cells into luteal cells that synthesize and secrete progesterone as well as estrogen. Estrogen is responsible for the development of the secondary sexual characteristics and drives the regeneration of the endometrium after menstruation and stimulates the proliferation of the uterine glands. Progesterone is released by the corpus luteum. Together with estrogen, it prepares the uterus for implantation, stimulates uterine gland secretion, and maintains the uterus during pregnancy. If pregnancy occurs, the placenta will eventually take over the production of both these hormones.

The Uterus

The wall of the uterus consists of three layers, the endometrium (the mucosa), the myometrium (muscular layer), and perimetrium (adventitial and serosal layer) (**Part C**). Primary functions of the uterus are to receive and maintain the embryo during pregnancy (primary function of the endometrium) and to expel the fetus at partuition (primary function of the myometrium). The endometrium contains uterine glands that secrete nutrients required to maintain the developing embryo during early implantation. The endometrium undergoes five different phases of transformation during the average 28-day menstrual cycle.

Phases of the Menstrual Cycle

From puberty to menopause, the endometrial layer undergoes cyclic changes that recur approximately every 28 days. This is referred to as the menstrual cycle. The first day of the menstrual cycle is marked by the onset of menstruation (sloughing of the endometrium). Even before the menstrual phase (days 1–5) is finished, the endometrial mucosa begins re-epithelializing. At this point in the cycle, serum levels of estrogen, progesterone, and LH are at their lowest level (**Part B**). With the release of GnRH from the hypothalamus, the anterior pituitary secretes FSH and serum levels of FSH increase. FSH stimulates some primordial follicles in the ovary to develop, beginning the proliferative (estrogenal) phase (days 6–14). In response to FSH, the follicle cells surrounding the oocyte begin secreting estrogen that stimulates the regeneration and growth of the endometrial mucosa (**Part C**). During this phase, the endometrium doubles its thickness, new coiled arteries grow into this layer, and uterine glands proliferate and accumulate within the mucosa. During most of this phase, estrogen has a negative feedback effect on the release FSH (via the hypothamus) but just prior to ovulation, this inhibitory effect is lost, causing a rapid rise in both FSH and LH. Meanwhile, a few of the stimulated follicles have progressed to the graafian follicle stage, and the few graafian follicles that remain complete meiosis I and begin meiosis II.

When both FSH and LH peak on day 13 or 14 of the menstrual cycle, ovulation occurs, and usually only one ovum is released. LH transforms the remaining follicle cells into a corpus luteum. The corpus luteum begins to synthesize and secrete progesterone in addition to estrogen. This is the secretory (progesteronal) phase (days 15–27). In response to the progesterone, the uterine glands begin secreting nutrients essential to implanting and maintaining the embryo. During this period, FSH and LH levels decrease. Implantation usually occurs about day 20–21 of the menstrual cycle. If pregnancy does not occur, the corpus luteum degenerates, dropping the serum levels of progesterone and estrogen (about day 27). This sudden decrease in progesterone and estrogen causes the coiled arteries within the endometrium to constrict, leading to ischemia in the endometrium. As a result, the menstrual phase begins. At this point, the luminal two thirds of the endometrium begins to slough off due to necrosis. The coiled arteries then relax and lose their constricted state and blood passes into the uteral lumen. Approximately 25–80 ml of blood are lost on average during this phase. Eventually the bleeding stops as clots form. Meanwhile, the corpus luteum slowly transforms into a corpus albicans. Should pregnancy occur, the implanting embryo releases hCG that maintains the corpus luteum until the placenta reaches a point of development where it can provide the progesterone and estrogen needed to maintain the pregnancy.

Clinical Aspects

While a typical menstrual cycle is described as 28 days long, the length of the menstrual cycle can vary greatly among normal women and may vary monthly in the same woman. Many factors, ranging from changing dietary and sleeping habits to stress, can alter the length of the cycle. Sometimes, a cycle is anovulatory (i.e., ovulation does not occur), and endometrial changes are minimal during such a cycle. The endometrium basically remains in the proliferative phase until menstruation occurs. An anovulatory state can also be induced artificially by administration of estrogen, with or without progesterone analogs, as is the case with birth control pills. These hormones are very effective in blocking ovulation because of their inhibitory effect on the secretion of GnRH needed for FSH and LH release. In addition to orally administered contraceptives, implantable subdermal slow-release carriers can deliver anti-ovulatory levels of hormones for 1–5 years. Induction of strong anti-progesteronal activity (i.e., RU-486 treatment) within 8 weeks of the last menstrual period will initiate menstrual sloughing of the conceptus along with endometrial decidua. Basal body temperature usually rises in response to LH near the time of ovulation. Because of this association, careful monitoring of body temperature is often used in the rhythm method of determining the ovulatory period.

4 Male Gametogenesis

A. Prepubescent Testis

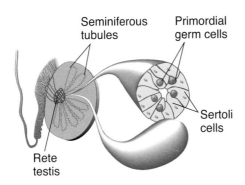

Seminiferous tubules

Primordial germ cells

Sertoli cells

Rete testis

B. Spermatogenesis
(puberty until death)

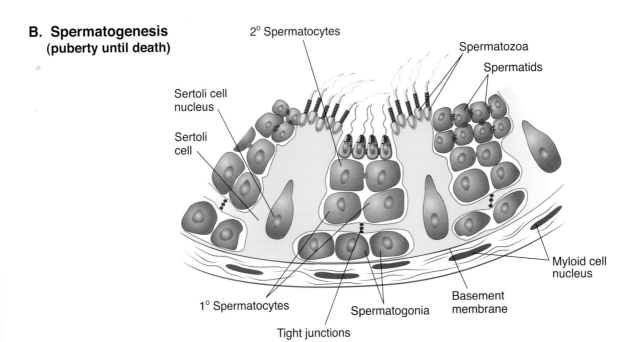

2° Spermatocytes

Spermatozoa

Spermatids

Sertoli cell nucleus

Sertoli cell

Myloid cell nucleus

1° Spermatocytes

Spermatogonia

Basement membrane

Tight junctions

C. Spermiogenesis

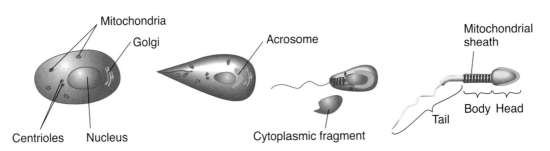

Mitochondria

Golgi

Acrosome

Mitochondrial sheath

Centrioles

Nucleus

Cytoplasmic fragment

Tail

Body Head

OVERVIEW

Male gametogenesis begins at puberty and continues until death. Prepubescent testes contain seminiferous tubules consisting only of Sertoli cells and primordial germ cells. At puberty under the influence of testosterone, primordial germ cells differentiate into spermatogonia, which undergo mitotic cell division. Some of the daughter cells of these spermatogonia differentiate into primary spermatocytes. Primary spermatocytes begin meiotic division. The second meiotic division produces spermatids, and spermatids transform into spermatozoa through a process called spermiogenesis. Spermatozoa must go through capacitation, the maturation steps essential for fertilization. To be fertile, men usually have sperm counts >10 million sperm/mL.

Male Gametogenesis

Differentiation of male primordial germ cells into spermatogonia begins at puberty. In the prepubescent testis, the seminiferous tubules are organized into closed 30–70 cm loops that anastomose at their ends. Each seminiferous tubule consists only of Sertoli cells and large primordial germ cells (**Part A**). At puberty, the primordial germ cells differentiate into spermatogonia under the influence of increased testosterone levels.

Spermatogenesis

The process of sperm production by mitotic cell division, meiosis, and cell differentiation is called *spermatogenesis*. Spermatogenesis begins at puberty and continues until death (**Part B**). Spermatogenesis occurs in synchronous waves along the seminiferous tubules, so one can find different stages along the length of individual tubules. During spermatogenesis, the developing germ cells remain deeply recessed into the Sertoli cell surface and remain connected to Sertoli cells while they develop into spermatozoa. The whole process of spermatogenesis takes about 64 days. During the sequence of cell divisions and maturation steps, the earliest stages of spermatogenesis are located closest to the periphery of the tubule, with the more mature cells located luminally.

Histologically, many stages of male gametogenesis can be observed in tissue sections of the adult testis (**Part B**). One can observe spermatogonia along the basement membrane of the seminiferous tubule. These cells are embryologically derived from the primordial germ cells and are the male gamete stem cell. Some daughter cells of the spermatogonia remain as spermatogonia, but others differentiate into primary spermatocytes. Primary spermatocytes undergo reduction division (meiosis I), forming 2 haploid gametes referred to as *secondary spermatocytes*. Secondary spermatocytes are difficult to find histologically because they very quickly undergo the second meiotic division to form spermatids. Interestingly, cell-cell separation between the daughter cells of primary and secondary spermatocytes is incomplete, and a thin bridge of cytoplasm interconnects them. Spermatids are haploid and have 1 representative strand of DNA for each chromosome (1n). At this stage, spermatids do not look anything like spermatozoa. Spermatids undergo a radical cellular transformation through a process called *spermiogenesis*. With respect to the sex chromosome content, 2 kinds of normal sperm are generated, those with an X-sex chromosome and those with a Y-sex chromosome.

Spermiogenesis

The transformation of spermatids into spermatozoa is called *spermiogenesis*. It is through this process that spermatids obtain the phenotypic characteristics associated with the spermatozoa (**Part C**). During this process the spermatid nucleus condenses, the microtubule-organizing center generates a flagellum, and much of the cytoplasm is lost. The Golgi apparatus of the spermatid is transformed into a vesicle called the *acrosome*, which tightly covers the end of the nucleus opposite the flagellum. The acrosome contains enzymes essential for the penetration of the ovum during fertilization. Other details about the transformation of spermatids into spermatozoa are beyond the scope of this text, but in the end the spermatids have a head with an acrosome-covered condensed nucleus, a midpiece region containing the flagellar base surrounded by energy-providing mitochondria, and a tail that provides motility. These odd-looking gametes (spermatozoa) are then released into the lumen of the seminiferous tubules, transported to the epididymis, and stored until ejaculation.

Capacitation

Spermatozoa, while they look morphologically mature, are functionally immature. A final maturation process called *capacitation* is required in order for spermatozoa to become metabolically active and attain their full capacity for fertilization. During this process, the spermatozoa undergo several modifications, including the acquisition of motility, changes in cell-surface proteins, and changes in acrosomal enzyme content. This process begins in the epididymis of the male reproductive tract and is completed in the female reproductive tract. Once in the female reproductive tract, human sperm usually do not survive longer than 24–72 hours.

Male Sterility

A normal ejaculate contains approximately 40–100 million spermatozoa/mL, but the spermatozoa constitute less than 10% of the ejaculate volume. The majority of the ejaculate consists of secretions from the seminal vesicles and the prostate and bulbourethral glands. In reproductively normal men, up to 20% of the spermatozoa in the ejaculate may be abnormal. Men with <10 million spermatozoa/mL are likely sterile, and the presence of abnormal or immobile sperm must be taken into account when assessing fertility. It is thought that one third to one half of the infertility cases in couples not practicing birth control stem from male infertility. Endocrine disorders, obstruction in the genital tracts, and abnormal spermatogenesis can render a male infertile. Environmental factors also may influence sperm counts. In experimental animals, abnormal sperm production increases with exposure to radiation, heat, pesticides, chemotherapy, drugs, carcinogens, and severe allergic reactions.

Sertoli cells are tightly interconnected to one another and form an immunological barrier (i.e., the blood-testis barrier) separating the spermatogonia in the basal compartment from the spermatocytes undergoing meiosis in the luminal compartment. How the primary spermatocytes are translocated to the luminal compartment is unclear, but cells undergoing meiosis in the male are immunologically different from those in the rest of the body and must be segregated. Autoimmune infertility can arise if this barrier is broken.

A. Fertilization

First polar body

Zona pellucida

Corona radiata cells

Maternal nucleus in meiosis II

Dispersal of corona radiata cells   1

Cortical granules

Acrosomal reaction (release of enzymes for penetrating zona pellucida)   2

Release of cortical granules

3

Fusion of plasma membranes

4

Penetration of sperm nucleus, initiation of zona (cortical) reaction, and completion of oocyte meiosis

D. Invading Blastocyst

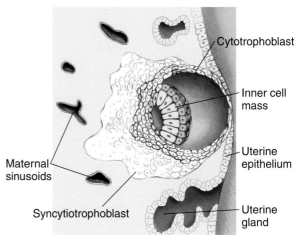

Cytotrophoblast

Inner cell mass

Uterine epithelium

Maternal sinusoids

Syncytiotrophoblast

Uterine gland

B. Fusion of Pronuclei

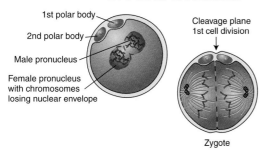

1st polar body

2nd polar body

Male pronucleus

Female pronucleus with chromosomes losing nuclear envelope

Cleavage plane 1st cell division

Zygote

E. Implantation   3   2   4

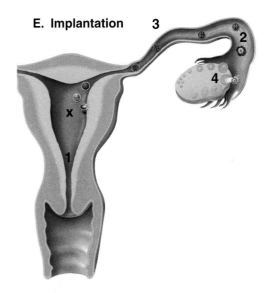

X

1

Implantation sites:
X. Normal, posterior wall of uterus
1. Internal os, (placenta previa)
2. Oviduct
3. Abdominal mesentery
4. Ovary

C. Early Zygote

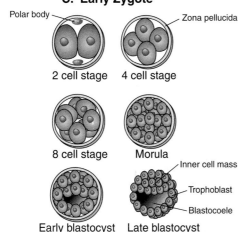

Polar body

Zona pellucida

2 cell stage   4 cell stage

8 cell stage   Morula

Inner cell mass

Trophoblast

Blastocoele

Early blastocyst   Late blastocyst

OVERVIEW

Fertilization of the ovum by spermatozoa restores the diploid number, determines the sex, and initiates cleavage and cell division. Fertilization occurs in several phases: (1) attachment of the spermatozoa to the zona pellucida; (2) penetration of the zona pellucida; (3) penetration of the oocyte plasma membrane and initiation of the cortical reaction; and (4) fusion of the 2 pronuclei and initiation of the first mitotic division. The zygote continues dividing, forming a solid ball of cells (a morula) and then develops into a fluid-filled blastocyst by the time it reaches the uterus. The blastocyst consists of an inner cell mass (future embryo) and an outer trophoblast layer (future conceptus portion of the placenta). The trophoblast is essential for the penetration and implantation of the conceptus into the uterine wall.

Fertilization

The ostium of the oviduct becomes closely apposed to the ovarian surface during ovulation, and the released ovum is usually swept into the oviduct. After insemination, spermatozoa swim into the uterus and up the oviducts, searching for the ovum. These spermatozoa remain viable for 1–3 days. Fertilization of the ovum usually occurs within the ampulla of the oviduct and takes about 12 hours to complete. Fertilization is usually divided into phases (**Part A**). First, spermatozoa penetrate the corona radiata, and then receptors on the spermatozoon bind specific glycoproteins within the zona pellucida. This triggers the acrosomal reaction. During the acrosomal phase, proteases released from the acrosome degrade the zona pellucida, facilitating penetration of the zona pellucida by the spermatozoon. The spermatozoon then attaches and fuses with the plasma membrane of the oocyte and then enters its cytoplasm. In response to the penetration, calcium quickly enters the ovum. This triggers the zona reaction whereby the contents of small vesicles (cortical granules) underlying the plasma membrane of the oocyte are released, making the membrane impermeable to other sperm. This prevents polyspermy (penetration by >1 sperm). Penetration of the spermatozoon also stimulates completion of the secondary meiotic division in the oocyte. The last phase of fertilization involves fusion of the pronuclei from the sperm and oocyte (**Part B**). As the 2 pronuclei are pulled together, each synthesizes DNA, the nuclear envelopes disappear, and the chromosomes align in the midline. At this point, the cell is referred to as a *zygote*. This is considered the zero time point of human development. The zygote completes mitosis, forming a 2-cell-stage zygote through a process known as *cleavage*. The size of the daughter cells actually decreases during subsequent cell divisions until the early blastocyst stage.

Morula and Blastula

As the zygote divides, it remains enveloped by the zona pellucida and within 3 or 4 days has grown to 16–32 cells. It is now referred to as a *morula* (**Part C**). As the cells divide, differential cell adhesion causes the exterior surface of the outer morula cells to become convexed and their interior surface to become concaved. This process is called *compaction* and results in the segregation of cells into 2 populations, the inner cell mass and outer cell mass. The morula then begins transporting fluids from the outside to the inside, forming a fluid-filled center called the *blastocyst cavity* (blastocoele), and causes the inner cell mass to become eccentrically placed. The zygote is now referred to as a *blastocyst* or *blastula*. The inner cell mass becomes the embryo proper (embryoblast) while the outer layer of cells forms placental membranes (trophoblast). The trophoblast releases degradative enzymes that break down the zona pellucida, and by the fifth or sixth day, the blastocyst "hatches" from the zona pellucida. At this point, the blastocyst usually has reached the uterus or is within the intrauterine portion of the oviduct. The trophoblast then differentiates into 2 cell types, the inner cytotrophoblast cells and the outer syncytiotrophoblast cells (**Part D**). The inner cytotrophoblasts are distinct mononuclear cells that undergo mitosis, and some

of these cells fuse to form the outer syncytiotrophoblast layer. The syncytiotrophoblast layer consists of a mass of indistinct, multinucleated cytoplasm that continues to grow by the addition of fusing cytotrophoblasts. Syncytiotrophoblasts synthesize hCG, progesterone, chorionic somatomammotropin, and other hormones required to maintain the pregnancy. Both cell types are responsible for generating the degradative enzymes needed for implantation.

Implantation

Implantation of the blastocyst usually begins on day 6 or 7 after fertilization. In response to the progesterone released from the corpus luteum, the endometrium becomes increasingly vascularized and edematous, and the uterine glands are activated. Upon contact with the blastocyst, the endometrium differentiates into highly metabolic, secretory cells that release growth factors and metabolites supporting implantation and early embryonic development. This endometrial reaction is called a *decidual reaction* and provides an immunologically privileged site for the blastocyst (an immunologically foreign body). The blastocyst releases degradative enzymes that permit it to invade the endometrium, and by day 9 it completely penetrates the endometrium (**Part D**).

Abnormal Implantation

The implantation site usually is found on the posterior wall of the body of the uterus. However, implantation may occur elsewhere and can lead to severe consequences (**Part E**). *Placenta previa* is a condition in which implantation occurs near the internal os (cervical opening) of the uterus. As the placenta develops, it covers the internal os and can cause severe bleeding during pregnancy and premature separation of the placenta from the uterus. Implantation outside the uterus is called an *ectopic pregnancy* and occurs with an incidence as high as 1/80 to 1/250 pregnancies. The most frequent causative factors are those that prevent movement of the zygote down the oviduct (e.g., pelvic inflammation), leading to tubal pregnancies (~90% of all ectopic pregnancies). Owing to the rich blood supply in the oviduct, the zygote can develop within the oviduct. Because the oviduct cannot accommodate a developing fetus, it often ruptures at 2–4 months of gestation. This is a life-threatening condition because of the high degree of hemorrhaging. It is often confused with appendicitis, particularly if it implants in the right oviduct. On rare occasions, implantation can occur on the surface of the ovary and is usually discovered through exploratory surgery for severe abdominal pain. Finally, implantation can occur within the abdominal cavity, generating symptoms similar to those of ovarian pregnancies.

Early Indications of Pregnancy

Indications of pregnancy include (1) the cessation of menstruation, (2) the presence of early pregnancy factor in the maternal serum (within 24–48 hours after fertilization), (3) the presence of hCG in maternal urine (detectable early in the second week), and (4) nausea and vomiting.

Fertility, Transgenics, and Cloning

A. In Vitro Fertilization and Embryo Transfer

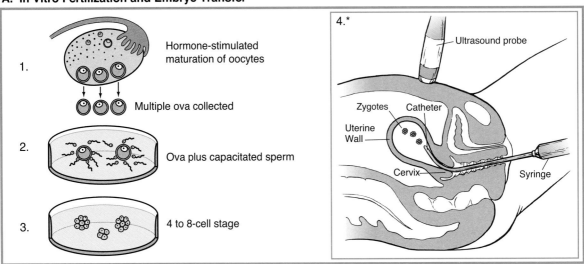

1. Hormone-stimulated maturation of oocytes

   Multiple ova collected

2. Ova plus capacitated sperm

3. 4 to 8-cell stage

4.*

Ultrasound probe

Zygotes   Catheter

Uterine Wall

Cervix

Syringe

B. Generation of Transgenic Mice from Embryo Stem Cells and Morula Cells*

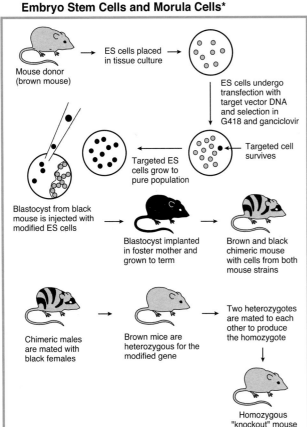

Mouse donor (brown mouse) → ES cells placed in tissue culture → ES cells undergo transfection with target vector DNA and selection in G418 and ganciclovir → Targeted cell survives

Targeted ES cells grow to pure population

Blastocyst from black mouse is injected with modified ES cells → Blastocyst implanted in foster mother and grown to term → Brown and black chimeric mouse with cells from both mouse strains

Chimeric males are mated with black females → Brown mice are heterozygous for the modified gene → Two heterozygotes are mated to each other to produce the homozygote

Homozygous "knockout" mouse

C. Cloning from Embryos

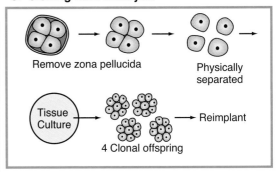

Remove zona pellucida   →   Physically separated

Tissue Culture   →   Reimplant

4 Clonal offspring

D. Cloning of Mammals from Adult DNA*

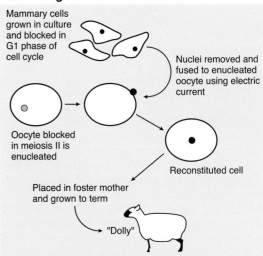

Mammary cells grown in culture and blocked in G1 phase of cell cycle

Nuclei removed and fused to enucleated oocyte using electric current

Oocyte blocked in meiosis II is enucleated

Reconstituted cell

Placed in foster mother and grown to term

"Dolly"

*From *Quick Look Genetics*, by Patricia Hoffer, 1999, with permission of Fence Creek Publishing, Inc., Madison, CT.

OVERVIEW

Fertility is the ability to reproduce. Sterility is the inability to reproduce owing to an inadequacy in structure or function. New technologies are available to circumvent many of the impediments to producing offspring. Animals having modified genes stably integrated into their genome cell are called transgenic animals. Once in the genome, these genes can be passed from generation to generaton. To make transgenic animals, genetically modified embryonic stem cells are implanted into the inner cell mass of early blastulae. These blastulae develop to form chimeric offspring with the modified cells incorporated through all adult tissues, including germ cells. Subsequent breeding of the heterozygotes generated from these chimeras is used to make homozygotes with the modification. These modifications also can include the removal of genes (knockouts). Transgenic animals are being used to generate animal models for studying normal biological processes and diseases.

In Vitro Fertilization and Infertility

Fertility is the ability to reproduce. *Sterility* is the inability to reproduce owing to an inadequacy in structure or function. Several methods are now available to circumvent sterility. In vitro fertilization and embryo transfer are often used in cases of sterility due to occlusion of the oviduct (**Part A**). First, ovulation is stimulated using hormones, and the ova are collected laparoscopically. Then the ova are combined with capacitated spermatozoa and fertilized within a petri dish, cultured until they reach the 4–8-cell morula stage, and then implanted into the uterus of the mother. This procedure, first performed over 30 years ago, has been performed successfully thousands of times. Resulting morulas can also be preserved a long time by freezing and then implanted after they are thawed. Some women can produce normal mature ova but are unable to maintain the pregnancy (e.g., no uterus because of a partial hysterectomy). For these women, ova can be collected laparoscopically, fertilized in vitro, cultured, and then implanted into a surrogate mother. Male sterility may stem from a low sperm count. Alternatively, spermatozoa may be unable to penetrate the zona pellucida and ova membrane, in which case a spermatozoon is directly microinjected into the cytoplasm of a mature egg in a process called *intracytoplasmic sperm injections*. Various in vitro techniques are being developed and refined to preselect the sex of the offspring. These include separating the X chromosome-containing sperm from the Y chromosome-containing sperm by their differing swimming abilities and morphologies and then using them in artificial insemination. The timing of sexual intercourse also can influence the sex of the offspring. Chances are more favorable for generating a male offspring if intercourse occurs 1–2 days after ovulation compared to near ovulation.

Chimeras and Transgenics

Each individual cell of a morula, if separated and implanted, is capable of forming an entire new individual that would be an exact genetic replica and contain the full complement of cell and tissue types. Cells capable of generating the entire spectrum of cell diversity found in an individual are said to be *totipotent*. One can also physically combine 2 separate morulas, making a giant morula that develops into a normal adult of normal size. This individual would contain 2 genetically different groups of cells and would be called a *chimera*. Cells representing each morula would be found within the inner cell mass and trophoblast. A chimera also can be produced by injecting a single morula cell into the inner cell mass of an early blastula. In that case, descendants of the transplanted cells would be found only in the early embryoblast and not in the trophoblast. This individual would still be a chimera, and daughter cells of the injected cell would be incorporated into all organ and tissue types found in the adult, including germ cells in the gonads. However, by the late blastula stage, cells have become more specialized and restricted in their developmental potential. The ability to introduce modified cells into an embryoblast that contribute to all the possible cell types in the adult is the basis behind generating transgenic animals.

Over the past 25 years or so, advances in cancer research, cell differentiation, and embryology have led to the isolation, development, and cell culture of particular cell lines that can be manipulated genetically and yet retain totipotency. These cells are called *embryonic stem (ES) cells*. ES cells or genetically modified ES cells can be injected into normal blastulae to form chimeric embryos that, when implanted into foster mothers, will form new individuals (**Part B**). Some cells in all the tissues of the individual, including the germ cells, are of ES cell origin. When these chimeras are mated with other normal individuals, a subset of the offspring will be heterozygotic for the introduced modified gene. When two heterozygotes containing the modified gene are crossed, a homozygotic individual with the modified gene is generated. Using this technology, researchers can generate animals that contain an artificially altered version of specific genes or that have a particular gene removed or disrupted (knockouts). These transgenic animals are now extensively used in the exploration of various effects that genetic mutations have on metabolic processes, embryonic development, and immunity, as well as in the generation of new biological assays and animal models. Some animals exhibit gain of gene function, loss of gene function, conditional expression of genetic mutations, or contain markers of gene expression.

Cloning

Physically separating morula cells, implanting them separately, and allowing them to develop represents "embryo cloning" (**Part C**). This resembles the process of forming identical twins through separation of the early zygote into 2 separate cells. Embryo cloning is different from the cloning of an individual using well-differentiated adult cells. Cloning an individual using the nuclear DNA obtained from a specialized adult cell involves nuclear transfer technology (**Part D**). With nuclear transfer technology, the nucleus of an adult differentiated cell is implanted into a denucleated egg. Under appropriate conditions, the adult DNA in this environment is reprogrammed so that previously irreversible changes in the DNA that made the cell differentiate are now capable of re-expression, and the cell undergoes development as if it were a normal zygote. While many species have been "embryonically cloned," only recently has it been possible to clone a mammal using DNA taken from adult specialized cells. However, the efficiency of this method is still very low.

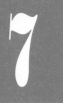

The Inner Cell Mass and Trophoblast

A. Blastula Development

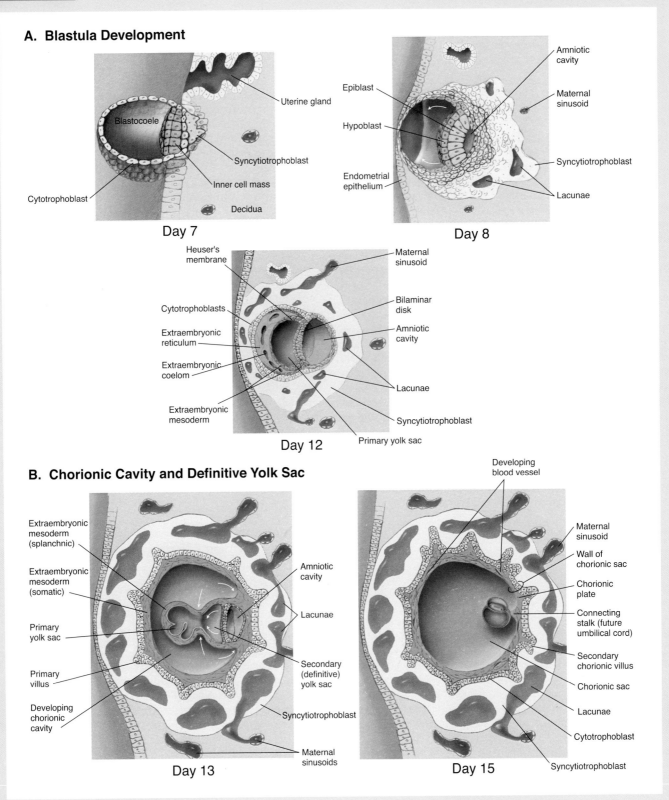

Day 7

- Uterine gland
- Blastocoele
- Syncytiotrophoblast
- Inner cell mass
- Cytotrophoblast
- Decidua

Day 8

- Amniotic cavity
- Maternal sinusoid
- Epiblast
- Hypoblast
- Endometrial epithelium
- Syncytiotrophoblast
- Lacunae

Day 12

- Heuser's membrane
- Cytotrophoblasts
- Extraembryonic reticulum
- Extraembryonic coelom
- Extraembryonic mesoderm
- Maternal sinusoid
- Bilaminar disk
- Amniotic cavity
- Lacunae
- Syncytiotrophoblast
- Primary yolk sac

B. Chorionic Cavity and Definitive Yolk Sac

Day 13

- Extraembryonic mesoderm (splanchnic)
- Extraembryonic mesoderm (somatic)
- Primary yolk sac
- Primary villus
- Developing chorionic cavity
- Amniotic cavity
- Lacunae
- Secondary (definitive) yolk sac
- Syncytiotrophoblast
- Maternal sinusoids

Day 15

- Developing blood vessel
- Maternal sinusoid
- Wall of chorionic sac
- Chorionic plate
- Connecting stalk (future umbilical cord)
- Secondary chorionic villus
- Chorionic sac
- Lacunae
- Cytotrophoblast
- Syncytiotrophoblast

OVERVIEW

The inner cell mass reorganizes into a bilaminar disk consisting of an epiblast and hypoblast. A new cavity develops within the epiblast layer (the amniotic cavity), while cells of the hypoblast migrate and line the blastocyst cavity (now the primitive yolk sac). The primitive yolk sac is replaced by a subsequent migration of hypoblast cells, forming the definitive yolk sac. New tissue, called extraembryonic mesoderm, develops between the definitive yolk sac and trophoblast layer. This mesoderm subsequently splits into two layers as the chorionic cavity forms. Meanwhile, the trophoblast differentiates into two cell types, the syncytiotrophoblasts and cytotrophoblasts. Cavities (lacunae) develop within the syncytial layer. As the blastocyst penetrates the endometrium, it erodes the maternal sinusoids, filling the lacunae with maternal blood and thereby establishing a primitive uteroplacental circulation.

Further Development of the Blastocyst

At 7 or 8 days of development, the inner cell mass reorganizes to form a bilaminar disk (**Part A**). Columnar cells adjacent to the cytotrophoblast layer comprise the epiblast, whereas the cells of the disk facing the blastocyst cavity comprise the hypoblast. A new cavity (the amniotic cavity) forms between the cytotrophoblasts and epiblast cells. Eventually, epiblast cells line this entire cavity. Epiblast cells lining the roof of the amniotic cavitry are referred to as amnioblasts. Meanwhile, the hypoblast cells migrate and form a thin cellular membrane (exocoelomic or Heuser's membrane) lining the original blastocyst cavity (now called the *primitive yolk sac*). A loose, acellular extracellular matrix (extraembryonic reticulum) is soon deposited between Heuser's membrane and the cytotrophoblast layer. A new population of cells then forms between the cytotrophoblasts and Heuser's membrane and migrates into this extracellular matrix as well as into the amnion region. This new tissue is called *extraembryonic mesoderm*. Eventually this new mesoderm splits with the one covering Heuser's membrane, called the *extraembryonic splanchnopleuric mesoderm,* and the other covering the cytotrophoblast and amnion, called the *extraembryonic somatopleuric mesoderm*. At the same time, spaces form within the remaining extraembryonic reticulum and coalesce, creating a large cavity known as the *extraembryonic coelom* or *chorionic cavity*. This cavity enlarges to the point that the developing embryo remains attached to the outer wall by only a stalk of mesoderm (future umbilical cord). Extraembryonic mesoderm lining the inner wall of the cytotrophoblast is known as the *chorionic plate*. Meanwhile, a second wave of cell migration from the hypoblast forms the secondary (definitive) yolk sac. As these cells migrate, they push Heuser's membrane away from the bilaminar disk. Because the

extraembryonic coelom is expanding at the same time, the primitive yolk sac is pinched off from the secondary yolk sac and eventually disintegrates. Embryonic mesoderm surrounding the definitive yolk sac is the initial site of hematopoeisis (blood formation) and blood vessel formation in the embryo.

Further Development of Trophoblast

By day 9, the expanding trophoblast layer forms large vacuoles (trophoblastic lacunae) as it extends into the endometrium. As the syncytium of the trophoblast invades the endometrium, it erodes and penetrates maternal sinusoids, spilling maternal blood into the lacunae. As the lacunae coalesce, maternal blood begins to flow through them and there is an exchange of oxygen, carbon dioxide, and nutrients, establishing the uteroplacental circulation at about days 11–13 (**Part B**). Maternal blood within the lacunae also acquires hCG synthesized by the syncytiotrophoblasts and cytotrophoblasts; this hormone is responsbile for maintaining the corpus luteum beyond its usual 14-day lifespan in the menstrual cycle. As the lacunae and sinuses enlarge, cytotrophoblasts covered with syncytiotrophoblast cells project into the lacunae, forming primary villi. These villi increase the surface area exposed to maternal blood. Eventually, the extraembryonic mesoderm penetrates the villi (secondary villi), and by the third week, blood islands and capillaries form within this mesoderm (tertiary villi). These capillaries eventually join those forming in the chorionic plate and connecting stalk. Some of the cytotrophoblastic tissue protrudes across the lacunae, penetrates the outer syncytial layer, and reaches the maternal endometrium. This tissue then forms a thin outer shell called the *outer cytotrophoblastic shell* (see also Chapter 41).

Gastrulation

A. The Primitive Streak

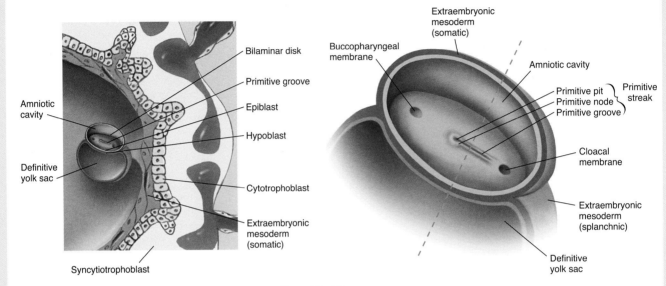

Bilaminar disk

Primitive groove

Epiblast

Hypoblast

Amniotic cavity

Definitive yolk sac

Cytotrophoblast

Extraembryonic mesoderm (somatic)

Syncytiotrophoblast

Extraembryonic mesoderm (somatic)

Buccopharyngeal membrane

Amniotic cavity

Primitive pit
Primitive node   } Primitive streak
Primitive groove

Cloacal membrane

Extraembryonic mesoderm (splanchnic)

Definitive yolk sac

Day 15-16

B. Gastrulation

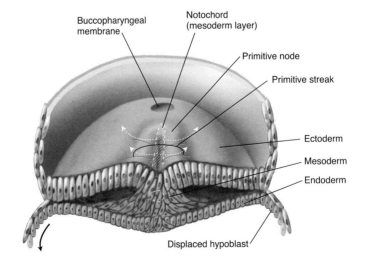

Buccopharyngeal membrane

Notochord (mesoderm layer)

Primitive node

Primitive streak

Ectoderm

Mesoderm

Endoderm

Displaced hypoblast

Day 15-16

OVERVIEW

The inner cell mass reorganizes into a bilaminar disk and then transforms into a trilaminar disk consisting of the ectoderm, mesoderm, and endoderm through a process called gastrulation. This is the start of the embryonic period. During gastrulation, intraembyronic mesoderm fills the space between the ectoderm and endoderm, except at the buccopharyngeal and cloacal membranes. A rod of mesoderm cranial to the primitive streak forms the notochord, a structure that induces the overlying ectoderm to differentiate into the neural plate. Perturbations in development before the beginning of the embryonic period usually lead to spontaneous abortion.

Embryonic Period

The pre-embryonic period encompasses fertilization through the 14th day. By day 14, the primitive uteroplacental circulation has formed, and the inner cell mass consists of a bilaminar disk. Perturbations in development during the pre-embryonic period usually result in spontaneous abortion. The embryonic period begins about day 15 and continues through the eighth week. It is the period when the trilaminar disk is formed and the 3 germ layers are transformed into the tissues and organs. By the end of this period, all the major organ systems have been established, and the embryo takes on a human shape. Therefore, the embryonic period is also known as the *period of organogenesis,* and it is during this period the embryo is most susceptible to factors interfering with development (e.g., teratogens).

Gastrulation

By day 15, the embryo consists of an epiblast and hypoblast layer. Beginning on day 15, an elongated groove (primitive groove) forms in the epiblast layer (**Part A**). By day 16, a deeper depression (the primitive pit) forms at the cranial end of the groove that is surrounded by a mound of cells (the primitive node). Together the node, pit, and groove make up the primitive streak. Formation of the primitive streak establishes both the longitudinal axis and right and left sidedness of the embryo. As the primitive streak forms, some of epiblast cells begin to delaminate and migrate from the base of the primitive groove and displace the hypoblast layer, forming the definitive endoderm (**Part B**). The delaminating cells (mesoblasts) then begin to migrate between the epiblast and the endoderm, forming the intraembryonic mesoderm. As cells continue to delaminate, epiblast cells keep moving toward the midline to fill the void. The intraembryonic mesoderm expands and becomes continuous with the extraembryonic mesoderm that covers the yolk sac and amnion. Eventually, the intraembryonic mesoderm intervenes between the entire ectoderm and the endoderm except at the site of the future mouth (the buccopharyngeal or oropharyngeal membrane) and at the site of the future anus (cloacal membrane). Here, the endoderm and ectoderm are fused but will eventually rupture, forming the oral and anal openings, respectively. The intraembryonic mesodermal cells also migrate anterior to the buccopharyngeal membrane, where they form precardiac mesoderm and mesoderm of the septum transversum. The cells remaining in the epiblast after gastrulation form the ectoderm.

Another group of invaginating cells migrates cranially from the primitive node, forming a mass of condensed mesoderm called the *notochord.* The notochord plays an essential role in the induction of the nervous system and in the transformation of some paraxial mesoderm into vertebral bodies. At about day 20, the primitive streak produces one last midline mass of mesoderm at the caudal end of the embryo called the *caudal eminence.* The structure is thought to contribute to caudal mesodermal structures and form the caudal-most portion of the neural tube. Once gastrulation is complete, the primitive streak quickly regresses. Later in development, the notochord regresses, with some remnants contributing to the nucleus pulposus of vertebrae.

Clinical Aspects

Sometimes the primitive streak does not regress fully, and persistent remnants develop into fast-growing sacrococcygeal teratomas. These tumors can become malignant in infancy and consist of tissues representing derivatives from all 3 germ layers. Occasionally, remnants of the notochord give rise to chordomas, slow-growing metastatic tumors that can infiltrate bone and are difficult to remove surgically. These patients often have a poor long-term prognosis (survival < 5 years). A wide spectrum of caudal dysplasias, including abnormal lumbar and sacral vertebrae, abnormal rotation of extremities (sirenomelia), and agenesis of urinary and reproductive organs, has been described. While their etiologies are unknown, they may involve abnormal function, migration, and proliferation of the caudal mesoderm during gastrulation.

9 Basic Body Plan I: Ectoderm and Neurulation

A. Neurulation

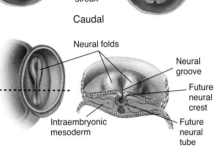

Cranial

Neural fold
Cut edge of amnion
Neural plate
Neural groove
Primitive pit
Primitive streak

Caudal

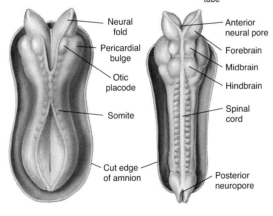

Neural folds
Neural groove
Future neural crest
Future neural tube
Intraembryonic mesoderm

Neural fold
Pericardial bulge
Otic placode
Somite
Cut edge of amnion

Anterior neural pore
Forebrain
Midbrain
Hindbrain
Spinal cord
Posterior neuropore

B. Neural Crest Formation

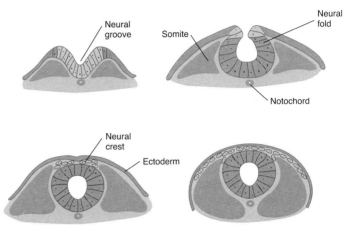

Neural groove
Somite
Neural fold
Notochord

Neural crest
Ectoderm

C. Major Neural Crest Derivatives

Cranial Neural Crest
Postganglionic parasympathetic neurons of ciliary, sphenopalatine, submandibular, and sublingual ganglia; peripheral ganglia of cranial nerves V, VII, IX and X.
Bones, cartilage, and odontoblasts of the maxilla and mandible; dermis and fat of the nose, face, middle ear, and neck; cranial vault bones; connective tissue of the thyroid, parathyroid, and anterior pituitary glands and lymphoid organs including the thymus and tonsils.
Vascular smooth muscle of great vessels and muscles of iris and ciliary body.
Aorticopulmonary and ventricular septation and cardiac innervation.

Trunk Neural Crest
Dorsal root ganglia.
Postganglionic parasympathetic neurons of viscera.
Postganglionic sympathetic neurons; chromaffin cells of adrenal medulla.

Other Neural Crest
Melanocytes, Schwann cells, pia and arachnoid of the forebrain and partial midbrain, carotid body, and parafollicular C cells of thyroid.

D. Major Neurocristopathies

Congenital Defects Involving Neural Crest Cells
Aorticopulmonary and ventricular septal defects
Hirschsprung's disease
Cleft lip and cleft palate
Craniofacial dysplasias
DiGeorge syndrome
Waardenburg's syndrome
CHARGE syndrome - coloboma (abnormal iris), heart defects, atresia of nasal conchae, retardation of development, genital hypoplasia in males, and abnormalities of the ear.

Tumors and Proliferation Defects in Neural Crest - Derived Cells
Neurofibromatosis (von Recklinghausen's disease)
Neuroblastoma
Pheochromocytoma

E. Neural Tube Defects

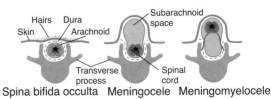

Hairs
Skin
Dura
Arachnoid
Subarachnoid space
Transverse process
Spinal cord

Spina bifida occulta   Meningocele   Meningomyelocele

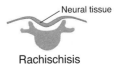

Neural tissue

Rachischisis

OVERVIEW

During gastrulation, the growing notochord induces formation of the neural plate from ectoderm. This plate flexes along the midline axis, forming 2 folds that rise and fuse in the middle to form the neural tube. This ectodermally derived neural tube eventually forms the brain and spinal cord. Incomplete closure of the neural folds leads to neural tube defects (NTDs), including anencephaly and myeloschisis. Tissue interactions between the neural tube and surrounding mesoderm induce the formation of vertebral arches. Improper development of vertebral arches leads to spina bifida, which may be accompanied by an overlying skin-covered cavity containing herniated meninges or neural tissue. Neural crest cells form at the site of neural fold fusion, and this migrating population of cells is important in the development of many different organs. Congenital defects and pathologies associated with defective morphogenesis of neural crest cells are called neurocristopathies.

Formation of the Neural Plate

During gastrulation, the developing notochord induces the overlying ectoderm to differentiate into tall columnar cells and form the neural plate (**Parts A** and **B**). This process begins at the cephalic end and progresses toward the primitive streak and historically is referred to as *primary induction.* As the notochord elongates, the neural plate broadens and eventually extends cranially up to the buccopharyngeal membrane. Formation of the neural plate is the first stage of neurulation.

Neurulation

On about day 22, the cephalic end of the neural plate begins to flex ventrally, forming a longitudinal midline groove (**Parts A** and **B**). Meanwhile, the lateral ends of the neural plate begin to elevate, forming 2 folds on either side of the neural groove. These neural folds continue to elevate, and their dorsal tips eventually meet in the midline and fuse. This forms a hollow cylinder called the *neural tube* and encloses a space called the *neural canal.* As the neural tube separates from the ectoderm, the overlying ectoderm reseals. Fusion of the neural folds begins on day 22 at the cervical level and progresses cranially and caudally. The neural tube will form the brain and spinal cord. Even before the neural folds close, specific regions of the future brain can be identified: the prosencephalon (forebrain), mesencephalon (midbrain), and rhombencephalon (hindbrain). Openings at the ends of the neural tube connecting the neural canal with the amniotic cavity are called the *anterior* and *posterior neuropores.* The anterior and posterior neuropores close by day 24 and day 26, respectively.

The Neural Crest

As the neural folds fuse, some of the cells at the fusion site separate and begin migrating away from the midline on either side of the forming neural tube (**Part B**). These new migrating cells are called *neural crest cells,* and they give rise to a large array of cell types that are instrumental in the formation of many organs. They first show up on about day 22 in the mesencephalon and then develop in a craniocaudal wave. The migration and differentiation of neural crest cells are influenced by their environment but also are restricted, in part based on the cranial or caudal axial level from which they arose. As seen in **Part C,** neural crest cells play instrumental roles in the development of several organ systems, the specifics of which are covered in subsequent chapters.

Neurocristopathies

Many congenital defects and pathologies are associated with defective morphogenesis of the neural crest cells. These are often referred to as *neurocristopathies.* A single defect or a whole spectrum of defects (a syndrome) may occur. A sample listing of neurocristopathies is found in **Part D**.

Abnormal Neurulation (NTDs)

Failure of the neural tube to close results in a multitude of congenital pathologies. The incidence of NTDs in newborns is about 1/1,000. Anencephaly (also known as craniorachischisis) results if the cranial neural folds fail to fuse and separate from the ectoderm or the anterior neuropore does not close. Affected individuals survive to the late fetal period or even to term but invariably die soon after birth. Rachischisis, or myeloschisis, occurs if caudal neural folds do not fuse and separate from the ectoderm (**Part E**). These individuals can survive but have significant clinical problems, depending on the extent of the anomaly. Failure of neural tube closure along the entire length of the embryo is called *craniorachischisis totalis* and leads to spontaneous abortion. Individuals with open neural tubes have elevated levels of α-fetoprotein in their amniotic fluid. Alpha-fetoprotein is a protein normally released into the lumen of closed neural tubes.

Etiology of NTDs

Nutritional and environmental factors play a role in the formation of NTDs. It is well documented that maternal dietary vitamin supplements (particularly folic acid) taken prior to conception and during pregnancy reduce the incidence of NTDs. Other drugs and agents taken during the first month of pregnancy increase the risk of NTDs.

Spina Bifida

As you will see in the next chapter, paraxial mesoderm surrounding the notochord and neural tube is responsible for forming the bone of the vertebral bodies and arches. Anomalies in the formation of the vertebral canal are referred to as *spina bifida* and may occur independent of any other spinal cord defect or as a consequence of failed neural tube closure (**Part E**). Spina bifida occulta is a condition whereby only a single vertebral arch fails to fuse while the neural tube and surrounding meninges develop normally. This missing vertebral arch usually occurs in the lumbar or sacral area. A tuft of hair, hemangioma, pigmented birthmark, or a dimple in the skin overlying the defect usually delineates the location of the defect. Spina bifida occulta is usually asymptomatic. In some cases of spina bifida, the contents of the vertebral canal bulge into a membrane-like, skin-covered cavity. Sometimes the dura and arachnoid protrude from the vertebral canal into these cavities, resulting in spina bifida with an accompanying meningocele. Spina bifida with a meningomyelocele involves a segment of the spinal cord or spinal nerve roots herniating into the cavity and is more common and severe than meningoceles. Meningomyeloceles and meningoceles may not be fatal but can cause severe life-long motor and mental impairments or impaired flow of cerebrospinal fluid (CSF), leading to swelling of the cerebral ventricles and hydrocephaly.

10 Basic Body Plan II: Intraembryonic Mesoderm

A. Intraembryonic Mesoderm Development

B. Sclerotome and Spinal Nerves

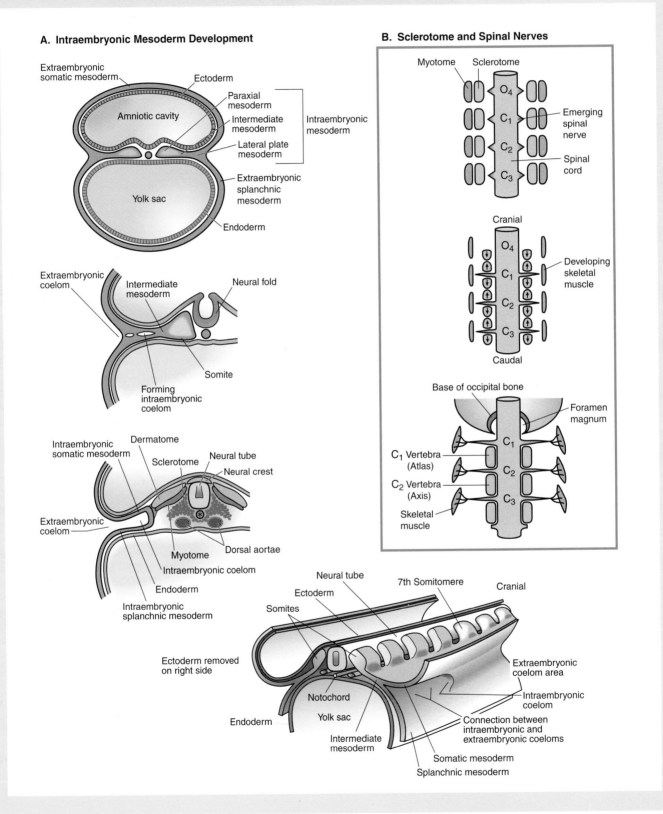

OVERVIEW

The intraembryonic mesoderm is arranged into 3 basic forms, the paraxial mesoderm, intermediate mesoderm, and lateral plate mesoderm. The paraxial mesoderm organizes into well-defined aggregates called *somites* and into loose cranial condensations called *somitomeres*. Somites reorganize further into the dermatome, myotome, and sclerotome. Somites contribute significantly to the axial skeleton, axial and limb musculature, and dermis. The major role of intermediate mesoderm is in the development of the urinary and genital system. Lateral plate mesoderm divides into intraembryonic somatic and splanchnic mesoderm, with the formation of an intervening cavity (the future body cavities). The somatic mesoderm contributes to the formation of the limb skeleton and connective tissue and to the walls of the body cavities. The splanchnic layer contributes to the formation of the cardiovascular system, walls of the visceral organs, and serosa.

Intraembryonic Mesoderm

The process of gastrulation leads to the formation of intraembryonic mesoderm (see Chapter 8). This mesoderm initially appears as a loosely organized, undifferentiated connective tissue, sometimes referred to as a *mesenchyme,* that becomes organized into 3 basic types (**Part A**). The paraxial mesoderm forms from mesoderm condensing on either side of the notochord, which then reorganizes into segmental condensations referred to as *somites* and *somitomeres* (see below).

The mesoderm immediately lateral to the paraxial mesoderm is referred to as the *intermediate mesoderm*. This mesoderm is important in the development of the urogenital organs and adrenal cortex; further development of this mesoderm is covered in later chapters.

The intraembryonic mesoderm lateral to the intermediate mesoderm is called the *lateral plate mesoderm* (**Part A**). This mesoderm is continuous with the extraembryonic mesoderm. Spaces form within this layer that coalesce to form tunnel-like cavities on either side of the embryo and connect to one another anterior to the buccopharyngeal membrane. This space is called the *intraembryonic coelom*. This space does not extend around the posterior end, but it does eventually open into the extraembryonic coelom at the midaxis level. The intraembryonic coelom is the primordium for the peritoneal, pleural, and pericardial cavities. The lateral plate mesoderm dorsal to the coelomic space and associated with the ectoderm is referred to as *intraembryonic somitic mesoderm* (somatopleure). It is continuous with the part of the extraembryonic mesoderm covering the amnion (i.e., extraembryonic somatopleure). Cells of the somatopleure lining the cavity will contribute to parietal peritoneum, parietal pleura, and parietal pericardium. This layer also will be a major contributor to the dermis of the body and limb mesenchyme. The lateral plate mesoderm ventral to the coelomic space and associated with the endoderm is called *intraembryonic splanchnic mesoderm* (splanchnopleure). This layer is continuous with the part of the extraembryonic mesoderm covering the yolk sac (i.e., extraembryonic splanchnopleure). Cells of the splanchnopleure will form not only the outer lining surface of the organs (differentiate into mesothelium and serous membranes, e.g., visceral pleura, visceral pericardium, and visceral peritoneum) but also the heart and walls of the viscera.

Somites

Paraxial mesoderm is the mesoderm found along either side of the notochord. It becomes organized into segmental structures called *somites* (**Part A**). Somites are tight and easily distinguishable aggregates of paraxial mesoderm that take on the general shape of a cube. The first pair of somites begins forming in the cervical region of the embryo at day 20, with additional pairs developing in a caudal direction until the end of the fifth week. There are 4 occipital, 8 cervical, 12 thoracic, 5 lumbar, 5 sacral, and 8–10 coccygeal somites. The first occipital and last 5–7 coccygeal somites eventually disappear. Cranial to the first somite, the paraxial mesoderm contributes to the formation of the facial muscles and muscles of the jaw and throat as well as to some of the bones of the skull. Data suggest that the cranial paraxial mesoderm is organized into 7 pairs of loose, indistinct, segmental condensations referred to as *somitomeres*.

Somite Differentiation

Each somite differentiates into 3 portions—the sclerotome, myotome, and dermatome (**Part A**). The most ventromedial part of the somite, the *sclerotome,* forms a migrating mesenchyme population that surrounds the notochord and neural tube. These cells eventually differentiate into bone and form the vertebral arches, vertebral bodies, and ribs. The dorsolateral part of the somite forms 2 layers, the dermatome and myotome. The dermatome contributes to the dermis underlying the skin in the neck, back, and sides. The remaining dermis of the body develops from the lateral plate mesoderm and neural crest cells. The myotome develops into the skeletal muscle for that particular axial segment. Some of the lateral-most myotomal cells migrate into the developing limbs, generating the limb musculature. More information about development of the appendicular skeleton and musculature is covered in Chapter 21.

Segmental Organization and Spinal Nerves

The spinal nerves develop segmentally and emigrate from the neural tube so that they emerge at same level as the corresponding somites. The sclerotomes of the somites form the vertebrae; hence, the developing vertebrae constitute a barrier to the emerging spinal nerves. This problem is circumvented because the sclerotome splits into cranial and caudal portions as the sclerotomal mesenchyme migrates toward the notochord (**Part B**). As sclerotomal mesenchymal cells migrate, the caudal group of cells join the preceding cranial group, and together they reorganize into intersegmental condensations. Seven cervical vertebrae form from 8 cervical somites because the cranial half of the first cervical sclerotome fuses with the caudal half of the fourth occipital somite to form the axis, and so on, resulting in 8 cervical nerves and 7 cervical vertebrae.

Clinical Aspects

Proper development of the sclerotome on both sides of the neural tube is necessary for normal vertebrae formation. If only one side fails, the resulting vertebra produces a serious form of scoliosis (lateral curvature of the spine). An extra rib is found in 0.5%–1% of the population, mostly at the seventh cervical level, where it can put pressure on the brachial plexus and subclavian artery.

Basic Body Plan III:
Endoderm and Early Body Folding

A. Endoderm Development and Body Folding

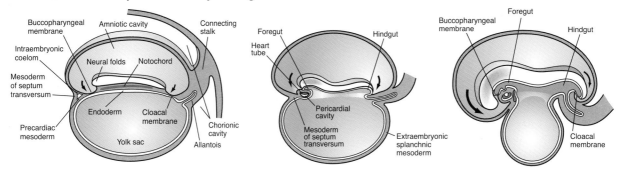

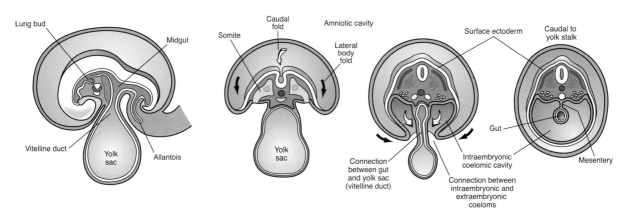

B. Body Cavities – Thorax from Abdomen

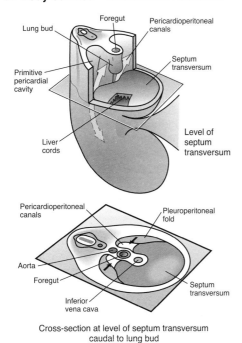

Cross-section at level of septum transversum
caudal to lung bud

C. Body Cavities - Pleural from Pericardial

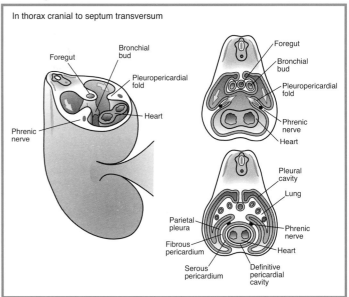

OVERVIEW

Body folding is driven by embryonic growth. As the neural tube lengthens, the embryo flexes along the cranial-caudal axis, pulling some endoderm inside to form the foregut and hindgut. At the same time, lateral body folds develop and fuse beneath the embryo, except at the midgut where the yolk sac protrudes outward. This separates much of the intraembryonic coelom from the extraembryonic coelom. The intraembryonic coelom forms the pericardial, pleural, and peritoneal cavities. As the cranial end of the embryo bends ventrally, the precardiac mesoderm and septum transversum swing beneath the foregut, partially separating the thoracic and peritoneal cavities. The septum transversum fuses with 2 pleuroperitoneal folds to form the diaphragm. Within the thoracic cavity, pleuropericardial membranes are carved from the thoracic wall and fuse in the midline, dividing the thoracic cavity into the pericardial and pleural cavities. Failure of the lateral body walls to fuse can lead to ectopic cordis and gastroschisis, whereas failure of diaphramatic closure can lead to life-threatening pulmonary defects.

Early Folding and Formation of the Early Gut

After gastrulation, the embryo is a relatively flat, 3-layered structure sitting above a large spherical yolk sac. From this, a cylindrical-like embryo forms, with a yolk sac and connecting stalk protruding from its midventral region. As the neural tube elongates, the embryo begins to bend and flex so that the head and tail ends curl beneath the main body of the embryo (**Part A**). This elongation and bending process pulls some of the endoderm of the yolk sac into the cranial and caudal ends of the embryo, forming the foregut and hindgut. Because of this, the embryo takes on a mushroom shape, with the yolk sac protruding from the midventral opening. This process also reverses the position of the precardiac mesoderm and septum transversum so that they now lie caudal to the buccopharyngeal membrane and ventral to the newly formed foregut. The part of the intraembryonic coelom once dorsal to the precardiac mesoderm (pericardial coelom) is now ventral to the precardiac mesoderm. A similar process occurs at the caudal end except that the connecting stalk of the embryo is pulled under the hindgut and cranial to the cloacal membrane.

As the embryo folds along the cranial-caudal axis, it develops lateral body folds that begin tucking beneath it. Eventually, these lateral body folds fuse, closing the connection between the intraembryonic and extraembryonic coeloms. This fusion begins at the cranial and caudal ends of the embryo and progresses toward the midventral part of the embryo, where the opening of the yolk sac is reduced to a narrow channel (the vitelline duct or yolk stalk). However, a narrow connection between the intraembryonic cavity (in the future peritoneal cavity) and extraembryonic cavity remains at the yolk stalk. This connection is eventually obliterated (see Chapters 15 and 41). As the lateral body folds unite, the overlying ectoderm and somatic mesoderm fuse with their counterparts to make a continuous seamless connection. The intraembryonic coelom, now within the embryonic body, will form the pericardial, pleural, and peritoneal cavities. As the lateral folds fuse, the portion of the amniotic cavity underlying the embryo expands, causing the connecting stalk and yolk stalk to be covered by the amniotic membrane. Together they form the primitive umbilical cord (see Chapter 41).

Primitive Mesenteries

As mentioned earlier, the lateral plate mesoderm splits to form the somatopleuric and splanchnopleuric mesoderm, with the intervening space generating the intraembryonic coelom. Once encased within the embryo body, cells from the somatic and splanchnic mesoderm lining the coelomic cavity differentiate into parietal and visceral serosa, respectively. Initially the gut is attached to the dorsal roof of the body wall by a broad segment of mesoderm, but as the gut develops, this splanchnic mesoderm narrows, eventually forming the dorsal mesentery (a doubled layer of visceral serosa from the splanchnic

mesoderm). A temporary ventral mesentery connecting the mesoderm of the gut to the outer body wall also forms, but it soon disappears except in the region of the stomach and developing liver. The somatic mesoderm under the ectoderm of the outer wall of the thorax, abdomen, and pelvis forms the body wall connective tissues and blood vessels.

Separation of the Body Cavity into Segments

The septum transversum, the plate of intraembryonic mesoderm that swung ventrally and caudally during cranial flexion, now occupies the space between the thorax and abdominal cavities (**Parts A** and **B**). The septum transversum does not completely close off these cavities, but the connection is reduced to 2 narrow canals on either side of the foregut called the *pericardioperitoneal canals* (**Part B**). During the fifth and sixth weeks, 2 new pleuroperitoneal membranes grow from the dorsal and lateral walls of the pericardioperitoneal canals, and these fuse with the septum transversum. This completely seals off the abdominal cavity from the thoracic cavity. Myoblasts from the septum transversum then invade the pleuroperitoneal membranes, forming the muscles of the diaphragm. The remaining cells of the septum transversum make the central tendon of the diaphragm. Folding and differential growth of the embryo cause the septum transversum to descend from its initial cervical position to the level of the future diaphragm. Because of its cervical origin, muscles derived from the septum transversum are innervated by the phrenic nerve (C3–5). However, a small portion of the diaphragm is derived from the body wall adjacent to the pleuroperitoneal membranes, and nerves from spinal levels T7–12 will innervate this muscle.

At about the same time the diaphragm is forming, 2 pleuropericardial folds form in the lateral walls of the thoracic cavity (**Part C**). These grow ventrally and medially and fuse with one another and the mesenchyme surrounding the foregut. The medial-ventral cavity is the definitive pericardial cavity and contains the developing heart, while the dorsal-lateral cavity becomes the pleural cavity.

Clinical Aspects

Occasionally during closure of the lateral body wall, the opposing body walls do not successfully fuse or enclose the thoracic or abdominal cavity. In the thorax, the heart may come to lie outside the thoracic cavity, causing a condition called *ectopic cordis*. Failure of the abdominal body walls to fuse can lead to gastroschisis (abdominal contents protrude from a fissure in the abdomen). Diaphragmatic hernias result as a consequence of incomplete fusion or hypoplasia of 1 or more of its constitutive components. This can lead to herniation of the stomach or intestines into the thoracic cavity (congenital diaphragmatic hernia). If the herniation of abdominal contents into the pleural cavity is extensive, it can lead to life-threatening pulmonary hypoplasia or an inablity to inflate the lungs.

12 Respiratory System (Lower Respiratory Tract)

A. Respiratory Primordia and Lung Bud Formation

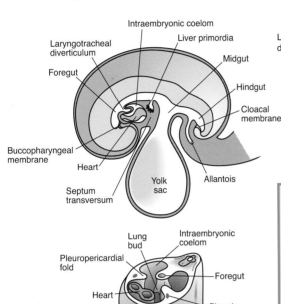

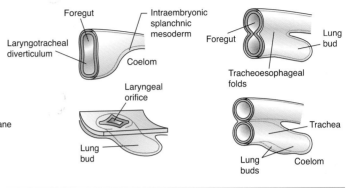

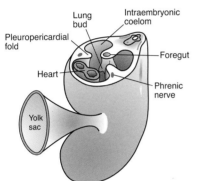

B. Branching Bronchial Buds

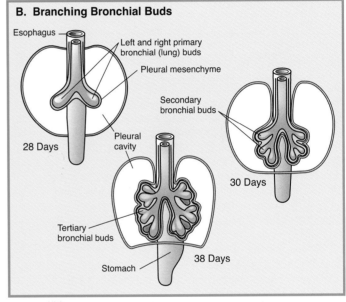

C. Development of Respiratory Epithelium

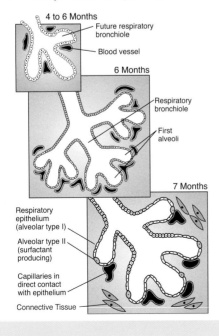

D. Tracheoesophageal Anomalies

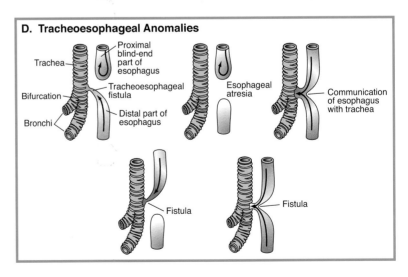

OVERVIEW

Stages of lung development can be divided into (1) the embryonic stage, during which the initial respiratory diverticulum and major bronchopulmonary segments are formed; (2) the pseudoglandular stage, when the branching pulmonary duct system reaches the terminal bronchiolar level; (3) the canalicular stage, when the respiratory bronchioles branch from the terminal bronchioles, with concomitant ingrowth of blood vessels surrounding these bronchioles; and (4) the terminal sac stage, when the alveoli buds form and alveolar type I and type II cells differentiate. Survival at birth requires that alveolar branching and surfactant secretion be progressed to a point that sufficient gaseous exchange occurs for sustaining life outside the womb. Respiration distress syndrome (hyaline membrane disease) occurs in approximately 2% of live births, particularly in premature infants, with a significant portion of them suffering from a surfactant deficiency. Tracheoesophageal fistulas, often accompanied by esophageal atresia, are the most common congenital anomaly found in the lower respiratory tract.

Initial Respiratory Primordia

The respiratory tract is composed of and includes the nasal cavity and oropharynx (the upper respiratory tract), and the larynx, trachea, primary bronchi, and lungs (the lower respiratory tract). The development of the upper respiratory tract is presented in Chapters 22 and 23. Development of the lower respiratory tract begins at about 4 weeks with the formation of a groove in the ventral floor of the posterior pharynx called the *laryngotracheal groove*. This endodermally lined groove deepens and forms a pouchlike diverticulum projecting into the splanchnic mesoderm called the *laryngotracheal diverticulum* (**Part A**). This elongated diverticulum becomes increasingly separated from the foregut by the development of longitudinal folds called *tracheoesophageal folds* (esophagotracheal ridges). These folds eventually fuse to form the tracheoesophageal septum, separating the foregut into a ventral laryngotracheal tube and a dorsal segment representing the future esophagus and oropharynx. While retaining an opening into the foregut via the laryngeal orifice, the laryngotracheal diverticulum elongates and together with the investing splanchnic mesoderm forms a lung bud. Therefore, the epithelium of the internal lining of the future larynx, trachea, bronchi, and alveoli is of endodermal origin, while the surrounding connective tissue and vasculature is derived from splanchnic mesoderm.

Larynx

Because of rapid proliferation of the splanchnic mesenchyme, the laryngeal orifice changes into a T-shaped structure. Meanwhile, the laryngeal epithelium proliferates rapidly and temporarily occludes the lumen, but it eventually recanalizes, forming the laryngeal ventricle and false and true vocal cords. The mesoderm in the fourth and sixth pharyngeal arches generates the cartilages and intrinsic muscles of the larynx. The laryngeal muscles, therefore, are innervated by the vagus nerve (cranial nerve X). Neural crest–derived mesenchyme surrounding this region forms laryngeal connective tissue.

The Lungs

The expanding lung bud bifurcates into 2 outpocketings called bronchial buds that grow and project into the pleuroperitoneal cavities (**Part B**). As each bronchial bud elongates, it continues to bifurcate, with the right bronchial bud dividing first into 3 main branches (the future secondary bronchi) and the left bronchial bud dividing into 2 main branches. This branching continues, forming smaller and smaller segments of bronchi until they reach the bronchiole level. Branching continues so that by 24 weeks about 17 or 18 generations of branching have occurred and terminal bronchioles have developed. However, some postnatal branching does occur. The epithelial lining of the terminal sacs formed at the ends of the terminal bronchioles consists of cuboidal epithelium but is eventually transformed into

thin and flattened squamous epithelial cells (**Part C**). These cells become increasingly associated with capillaries developing in the splanchnic mesoderm. Epithelial cells lining the terminal sacs (alveoli) differentiate into 2 cell types, alveolar type I cells and alveolar type II cells. Type I cells and capillary epithelium, together with the intervening extracellular matrix, will make up the blood-air barrier. At the beginning of the 24th week, alveolar type II cells begin to appear. These cells synthesize and secrete surfactant (ß-dipalmitoyl lecithin), a phosopholipid that lowers the surface tension at the air-alveolar interface. Levels of surfactant increase during the last 2 months of gestation. At birth, the lungs are almost half-filled with fluid from the amniotic cavity and derived from the lungs themselves. This fluid is removed rapidly at birth by transport into the pulmonary capillaries and lymphatics and by expulsion through the mouth and nose from increased thoracic pressure during vaginal delivery.

Respiratory Distress Syndrome

Respiratory distress syndrome (also known as hyaline membrane disease) accounts for approximately 25,000 deaths per year in the U.S. and is usually due to either insufficient surfactant or a neurological insufficiency (immature or poorly functioning respiratory brain center). The maturation of alveolar type II cells varies widely in fetuses, and even full-term babies can exhibit deficiencies in surfactant. The reasons for this are unclear, but it appears to be related in some way to hormones and growth factors. Glucocorticoid treatment during pregnancy accelerates fetal lung development, including surfactant production. Therefore, glucocorticoids have been used clinically to help prevent respiratory distress syndrome.

Other Congenital Anomalies

Tracheoesophageal fistulas result from an incomplete division of the foregut into respiratory and esophageal segments (**Part D**). It is the most common anomaly of the lower respiratory tract and is often accompanied by esophageal atresia. Infants with this anomaly cough, choke when they swallow, and regurgitate food. Hydramnios and polyhydramnios (excessive amniotic fluid) are often associated with esophageal atresia and tracheoesophageal fistulas because excessive amniotic fluid cannot pass into the fetal stomach and intestines where it is absorbed and transferred to the placenta for removal. For unknown reasons, tracheoesophageal fistulas and esophageal atresia are more prevalent in male infants than female infants. Abnormalities of the lung and bronchiolar tree are rare. Occasionally, however, an ectopic lung lobe may arise from the trachea or esophagus. Lung hypoplasia is characterized by a large reduction in lung volume. It often accompanies a congenital diaphramatic hernia whereby the abdominal contents abnormally occupy the thoracic cavity, restricting development and expansion of the lungs.

For each of the following questions, choose the **one best answer**.

1. When does ovulation occur during the menstrual cycle?

(A) It occurs when circulating levels of both FSH and LH are at their lowest.

(B) It occurs when there is a rapid fall in the serum levels of progesterone and estrogen.

(C) It occurs when the corpus luteum begins secreting progesterone.

(D) It occurs when the secretory phase ends.

(E) It occurs approximately 14 or 15 days after the onset of the last menstrual period.

2. A baby is born with multiple defects, including a heart defect, cleft lip and palate, and defects in facial skin pigmentation. What is the most likely common embryological basis for these defects?

(A) The process of gastrulation was abnormal.

(B) The migration and proliferation of neural crest cells were insufficient.

(C) Paraxial mesoderm cells failed to differentiate properly.

(D) There was hypoplasia of the cranial splanchnic mesoderm.

(E) The neural tube failed to close.

3. A newborn child exhibits severe lumbar scoliosis. What is the most likely embryological basis for this anomaly?

(A) Sclerotomal cells did not migrate and differentiate on one side of the lumbar neural tube.

(B) Neural crest cells did not form at this axial level.

(C) The neural tube did not close in the lumbar region.

(D) There was too much amniotic fluid.

(E) The notochord failed to develop in this region.

4. A couple desiring to conceive a child closely monitor the female's menstrual cycle and her changes in body temperature to best gauge the time for ovulation. Within what period of time after the release of the ovum would fertilization have to occur in order to produce a zygote?

(A) 1–2 hours

(B) 24 hours

(C) 2–3 days

(D) 3–5 days

(E) 6–7 days

5. A 28-year-old patient with a history of endometriosis enters the emergency room complaining of severe abdominal pain. Her last menstrual period was about 9 weeks ago, and tests indicate she is pregnant. Moreover, she is beginning to show signs of shock suggesting internal hemorrhaging and is rushed into emergency surgery. The surgeon stops the bleeding and removes her right uterine tube. What was the most likely diagnosis?

(A) Ovarian cyst

(B) Placental previa

(C) Ectopic pregnancy

(D) Pelvic inflammatory disease

(E) Implantation bleeding

6. A dietary deficiency of folic acid increases the risk of developing what kind of defects?

(A) NTDs

(B) Polyploidy

(C) Ambiguous genitalia

(D) Microdeletions in gametes

(E) Limb defects

7. If you were trying to design a contraceptive agent targeting the ability of spermatozoa to fertilize an ovum, what possible avenues could you take?

(A) Develop agents enhancing acrosomal enzyme synthesis during spermiogenesis

(B) Develop agents blocking the zona reaction

(C) Develop agents increasing mitochondrial energy production in spermatozoa

(D) Develop agents blocking the binding of spermatozoa cell-surface receptors to the zona pellucida

(E) Develop agents preventing calcium influx into the ovum when spermatozoa penetrate it

8. What cells are the male reproductive stem cells in the adult?

(A) Sertoli cells

(B) ES cells

(C) Spermatogonia

(D) Spermatocytes

(E) Primordial germ cells

9. What tissue or structure is responsible for synthesizing and secreting progesterone until the placenta can supply the progesterone needed for maintaining the pregnancy?

(A) Cytotrophoblasts

(B) Corpus luteum

(C) Syncytiotrophoblasts

(D) Graafian follicle

(E) Decidua

10. What hormone is measured in most home pregnancy tests?

(A) hCG

(B) Early pregnancy factor

(C) Progesterone

(D) Estrogen

(E) LH

11. A new arrival in the neonatal unit is fed for the first time but begins choking immediately. What is the most likely congenital reason for the choking response?

(A) Patent thyroglossal duct

(B) Pyloric stenosis

(C) Meckel's diverticulum

(D) Aganglionic colon

(E) Esophageal atresia

12. A newborn is extremely cyanotic and, even in the presence of 100% oxygen, soon dies. Autopsy results show that the diaphragm was incomplete, and the stomach and small intestine had herniated into and occupied much of the thoracic cavity. The lung developed but was severely hypoplastic. What is the most likely embryological basis for this defect?

(A) Formation or fusion of the pleuroperitoneal folds failed on the left side.

(B) There was abnormal lengthening of the small intestine.

(C) There were abnormal proliferation and branching of the respiratory epithelium.

(D) The infant had situs inversus.

(E) There was a congenital absence of the pericardium.

Questions 13 and 14.
A man and woman have been trying to conceive and produce a child for several years and, after being unsuccessful, sought help at a fertility clinic. The female patient had a history of endometriosis. Using endovaginal sonography, the physician discovered that both uterine tubes were obstructed. However, tests showed that she still produced ova and that the male produced sufficient normal spermatozoa.

13. Which of the following possible avenues of treatment might a physician suggest to the couple if they want to produce a child using their own gametes?

(A) Cloning

(B) Artificial insemination

(C) In vitro fertilization

(D) Gonadotropin therapy

(E) Pronuclear transfer

14. This treatment would mostly likely require which of the following techniques?

(A) Gonadotropin therapy

(B) Laparoscopy

(C) Tissue culture

(D) Artificial capacitation of spermatozoa

(E) Artificial implantation into a primed uterus

(F) All of the above

15. What is the fate of the outer cell mass of a blastula?

(A) It undergoes a decidua reaction.

(B) It forms the bilaminar disk.

(C) It forms the hypoblast.

(D) It forms the trophoblast.

(E) It regresses once implantation is complete.

16. What would happen if you were to take cells from one morula, inject them into the inner cell mass of an early blastula host, and then implant this blastula into a surrogate mother?

(A) The injected cells would be rejected and die; all the cells in the fetus would be from the host blastula.

(B) Some of the injected cells would be incorporated into the developing placenta of the fetus.

(C) Some of the primordial germ cells in the fetus would be derived from the injected morula cells.

(D) All cells in the fetus would be derived from the injected morula cells.

(E) The entire inner cell mass of the host would die and, if implanted, would result in a molar pregnancy.

17. A newborn has a large, skin-covered bulge (protrusion) at the posterior lower lumbar region. In addition, there is paralysis in the lower extremities. Closer examination using magnetic resonance imaging (MRI) shows that the cavity is lined by meninges and that the spinal nerves herniate into the cavity. What is your diagnosis?

(A) A meningocele

(B) A meningomyelocele

(C) A meningohydroencephocele

(D) Rachischisis

(E) Arnold-Chiari syndrome

18. One hour after birth, the respiratory rate of a normal-appearing newborn began increasing, eventually reaching a rate of 65–70/min. Breathing became labored, and auscultation of the chest revealed diminished air entry. Eventually the child became cyanotic and, even in the presence of 100% oxygen, died. Autopsy results revealed the lungs to be very red and fleshy in appearance and the alveoli collapsed tp be filled with eosinophils and covered with a membrane-like material. What is your diagnosis?

(A) Anaphylactic shock

(B) Tracheoesophageal fistula

(C) Diaphragmatic hernia

(D) Apnea

(E) Respiratory distress syndrome

19. What is the correct developmental sequence regarding the formation of the embryonic germ layers from the blastula?

(A) Inner cell mass → epiblast → mesoderm → endoderm

(B) Inner cell mass → epiblast → endoderm → mesoderm

(C) Outer cell mass → syncytiotrophoblast → cytotrophoblast → endoderm

(D) Inner cell mass → cytotrophoblast → hypoblast → ectoderm

(E) Outer cell mass → hypoblast → ectoderm → endoderm

20. What is the karyotype of an unfertilized ovum?

(A) Diploid and 2n

(B) Diploid and 4n

(C) Haploid and 2n

(D) Haploid and 1n

(E) Diploid and 1n

21. A baby is born with a distended abdomen because of a congenital absence of abdominal muscles (prune-belly syndrome). What is the most likely embryological basis for this anomaly?

(A) Myotomal cells failed to migrate and proliferate.

(B) Myoblast cells from the somitomeres degenerated.

(C) The apical epidermal ridge failed to develop.

(D) Neural crest cells failed to migrate and proliferate.

(E) None of the above.

Questions 22 and 23.

A female patient has a difficult time delivering an infant because of a large bulging mass of tissue in the posterior area of the infant's buttocks. After delivery, gentle rectal palpation indicated that this tissue extended up into the pelvis. Biopsy of the tissue revealed the presence of skin, cartilage, bone, nervous tissue, cardiac and skeletal muscle, and intestinal epithelium.

22. What is your diagnosis?

(A) Sacrococcygeal teratoma

(B) Teratocarcinoma

(C) Pheochromocytoma

(D) Choriocarcinoma

(E) Chordoma

23. What is the origin of this tumor?

(A) These tumor cells were derived from a molar pregnancy.

(B) These tumor cells came from remnants of the notochord.

(C) These tumor cells came from stray primordial germ cells.

(D) These tumor cells came from cells belonging to the primitive streak.

(E) These tumor cells came from remnants of the caudal eminence.

24. Which of the following regarding mitosis and meiosis is *true*?

(A) Cells initiating meiosis do not replicate their DNA.

(B) Like mitosis, meiosis only has a single metaphase step.

(C) Meiotic cells undergo synapsis while mitotic cells do not.

(D) When complete, mitotic cells are haploid.

(E) During mitosis and meiosis, paternal and maternal chromosomes are randomly segregated into the daughter cells.

Questions 25–27.
Match each of the descriptions with the most appropriate term.

(A) FSH

(B) LH

(C) Estrogen

(D) Progesterone

(E) hCG

25. Initiates follicle development. A

26. Stimulates the regrowth of the endometrium after the menstrual phase. C

27. Transforms the cells of the stratum granulosum into cells secreting the hormones needed to prepare the endometrium for implantation. B

ANSWERS

1. The answer is E.

Ovulation usually occurs in the middle of the menstrual cycle (day 14 or 15) when blood levels of FSH and LH suddenly surge. This surge initiates changes in the graafian follicle and ovary, leading to release of the ovum. After ovulation, the remnants of the graafian follicle are transformed into the corpus luteum. The corpus luteum secretes the progesterone and estrogen needed to prepare the uterus for implantation (the secretory phase). If implantation does not occur, the corpus luteum involutes after approximately 14 days, causing a rapid decrease in progesterone and estrogen levels and initiating menstruation.

2. The answer is B.

This spectrum of defects can occur as a consequence of abnormal morphogenesis of neural crest cells. Migration, proliferation, and differentiation of neural crest cells is necessary for generating the mesenchymal cells needed for cardiac septation and for forming the craniofacial primordia. Neural crest cells are also the progenitor cells for melanocytes found in the skin. Many other cell types and tissues

are derived from neural crest cells. Therefore, genetic or environmental factors targeting neural crest cell populations can lead to a broad range of congenital defects.

3. The answer is A.

Somites on either side of the neural tube segregate into a sclerotome, dermatome, and myotome. Sclerotomal cells migrate medially on both sides of the neural tube and notochord, where tissue-tissue interactions induce these cells to differentiate into bone, forming the vertebral bodies and vertebral arches. Improper tissue interactions resulting in unilateral failure of proliferation and differentiation of the sclerotome lead to severe scoliosis.

4. The answer is B.

After its release, the approximate lifespan of an ovum is 24 hours. In contrast, spermatozoa have a lifespan between 1–3 days within the female reproductive tract. If the ovum is not fertilized within that time-frame it degenerates as it moves down the oviduct.

5. The answer is C.

Both endometriosis and pelvic inflammatory disease often lead to the formation of obstructions or pockets within the uterine tubes (oviducts). While the smaller spermatozoa can make their way up the uterine tube and fertilize the ovum, the zygote often becomes lodged or its descent delayed within the uterine tube. Once the zygote reaches the blastula stage, it begins implanting, and if it is still within the uterine tube, it implants there. As the embryo continues to develop and grow, the uterine tube stretches to accommodate the embryo, leading to abdominal pain and cramping. However, the uterine tube reaches a point where it can no longer accommodate the developing embryo or fetus, and eventually the uterine tube ruptures. Because the uterine tube is richly vascularized, rupture of the uterine tube causes massive hemorrhaging that endangers the life of the patient.

6. The answer is A.

It is well documented that deficiencies in folic acid increase the risk of NTDs, including spina bifida and anencephaly. Moreover, there is an increased risk of developing various congenital neurocristopathies. Dietary supplementation before and during pregnancy greatly lowers the risk of these defects. While the mechanism through which folic acid works is unclear, studies suggest that it may be related to circulating levels of homocysteine, a normal metabolite found in serum.

7. The answer is D.

Binding of the spermatozoa to the zona pellucida of the ovum is essential for triggering the release of acrosomal enzymes, thereby facilitating penetration of the spermatozoa. Flagellar swimming requires energy provided by the mitochondria; therefore, a drug increasing mitochondrial energy production in spermatozoa might increase the capability of spermatozoa to penetrate the zona pellucida and reach the ovum.

8. The answer is C.

Primordial germ cells are the progenitors of both male and female reproductive stem cells. In the testes of prepubescent males, the seminiferous tubules consist of Sertoli cells (the support cells) and primordial germ cells. At puberty, these germ cells differentiate into spermatogonia, the male gamete stem cells. Spermatogonia continually divide, with one daughter cell eventually differentiating and producing the spermatocytes while the other daughter cell replaces the parent. In females, primordial germ cells differentiate into oogonia, the female gamete stem cell. Oogonia divide, and during the late embryonic or early fetal period they differentiate into oocytes and begin meiosis.

9. The answer is B.

The rapid increase in LH at the time of ovulation transforms the remnant of the graafian follicle into a corpus luteum, a temporary endocrine organ whose cells produce progesterone and estrogen. These latter 2 hormones are needed to prepare the uterus for implantation. However, the corpus luteum has a limited life span of approximately 14 days unless fertilization occurs and trophoblastic tissue is formed. Syncytiotropoblasts and cytotrophoblasts secrete hCG, and this extends the life of the corpus luteum until the placenta makes sufficient amounts by itself.

10. The answer is A.

hCG was the first hormone used in commercial, over-the-counter pregnancy test kits. It is still the most common one used because the test is easy to perform, it does not require invasive techniques (can be performed as a urine test), and the level of this hormone is usually high enough to detect within 2 weeks of fertilization (approximately the same time the woman suspects possible pregnancy due to a missed menstrual period). This hormone is secreted by the trophoblastic tissue of the implanting blastula. Measurement of early pregnancy factor requires a blood test but can detect pregnancy as early as 24 hours after fertilization.

11. The answer is E.

With esophageal atresia, the esophagus ends as a blind sac due to abnormal separation of the esophagus from the tracheal diverticulum. There are several variations of the defect, but many exhibit stenosis or atresia of the esophagus with or without a fistula between the esophagus and trachea. In this case, when fed milk, the infant regurgitated it almost immediately because of esophageal atresia and began choking on the regurgitated milk. It usually is surgically repaired.

12. The answer is A.

Failure of the pleuroperitoneal folds to form and subsequently fuse with the septum transversum leads to incomplete formation of the diaphragm. Consequently, the abdominal contents often herniate into the pleural cavity during embryonic and fetal development (congenital diaphragmatic hernia). This prevents normal pulmonary development, leading to pulmonary hypoplasia. The hernia can be repaired after birth, and the infant may have sufficient gaseous exchange to sustain life if the degree of hypoplasia is not too severe.

13 and 14. The answers are C and F, respectively.

In vitro fertilization is now routinely performed but requires that ova be collected from the female patient. The female patient would be treated with gonadotropins to induce follicle development and produce ova. These ova would then be aspirated using ovarian laparoscopy. Once collected, the ova would be combined in tissue culture with capacitated spermatozoa taken from the male patient. Once fertilized, the zygote would be cultured in vitro until it reached the 4–8-cell stage and then implanted into the uterus via a catheter passed through the vagina and os of the cervix. Previous hormonal therapy would be used to prepare the uterus for implantation. Many of the same techniques are used in situations in which the male spermatozoa are unable to penetrate the zona pellucida and ovum plasma membrane. In that situation, the male pronucleus is directly microinjected into the ova in vitro.

15. The answer is D.

The morula consists of an inner and outer group of cells, and once a blastula cavity develops, the inner group becomes eccentrically positioned and forms the inner cell mass. The outer layer differentiates into trophoblastic tissue and subsequently into cytotrophoblastic and syncytiotrophoblastic layers. The trophoblastic tissue is responsible for implantation and eventually forms the fetal portion of the placenta. The inner cell mass forms the embryo. The inner cell mass forms a bilaminar disk of cells that, through the process of gastrulation, makes all 3 embryonic germ layers of the embryo.

16. The answer is C.

Morula cells are totipotent and therefore capable of being incorporated and differentiating into any of the cells found in the fetus or placenta. The inner cell mass of an early blastula develops into the embryo while the outer cell mass (trophoblast) forms the placenta. Given that the cells were injected into the inner cell mass, the cells would contribute only to cells found in the embryo and fetus. This would include germ cells. Since the embryo does not have a functional immune system at this point, the cells would not be immunologically rejected. This procedure is commonly used to generate transgenic animals, but usually only a single cell is injected into the inner cell mass. It has also been performed with primates, and the technology has progressed to the point that it likely can be applied to humans as well.

17. The answer is B.

A meningomyelocele is a form of spina bifida whereby the vertebral arches are missing and a meningeal-lined cavity forms containing herniated spinal cord tissue. Because this type of defect impairs normal spinal cord development, it is often associated with neural deficits such as paralysis. Meningomyeloceles can occur anywhere along the vertebral column, but most commonly occur in the lumbar and sacral regions.

18. The answer is E.

The alveolar type II cells of this child were not mature enough or did not synthesize sufficient levels of surfactant to sustain life. Without surfactant, the surface tension between the air and moist alveolar type I cells is too great to permit efficient gaseous exchange or to permit the lungs to expand completely. In addition, the air may damage the lung epithelia in the absence of sufficient surfactant. Effusion of protein-containing fluids and eosinophils from the circulation into the alveolar sacs produces a glassy membrane-like substance (hyaline membrane) overlying the luminal side of the alveoli. This also reduces gaseous exchange. If the condition is severe enough, the infant will not be able to get the oxygen needed even if provided 100% oxygen. This condition is common in premature infants and newborns of diabetic mothers. Corticosteroid treatment during pregnancy accelerates fetal lung development and differentiation of alveolar type II cells. It is sometimes used to prevent respiratory distress syndrome.

19. The answer is B.

The inner cell mass forms a bilaminar disk that organizes into 2 layers, the epiblast and hypoblast. The hypoblast forms the primitive yolk sac. The epiblast develops a thickened area called the primitive streak and node, and this is the site of gastrulation. During early gastrulation, mesoblast cells delaminate from the epiblast, begin migrating, and first replace the hypoblast cells with the definitive endoderm. When nearly completed, the mesoblast cells then begin migrating between the endoderm and epiblast to form the intraembryonic mesoderm. After gastrulation is complete, the remaining epiblast is referred to as ectoderm. These 3 germ layers generate all the tissue and organs found in the embryo, fetus, and adult.

20. The answer is C.

Just prior to ovulation, the primary oocyte (which is diploid and 4n because of prior DNA synthesis) completes meiosis I. The secondary oocyte, now haploid and 2n, begins meiosis II without an intervening DNA synthesis step. However, it stops at metaphase II. The secondary oocyte remains in this state until fertilized. Therefore, the ovum is really a secondary oocyte that is haploid and 2n. Once a spermatozoon penetrates the ovum, the secondary oocyte completes meiosis II, forming a mature, haploid, 1n female gamete just before the female pronucleus fuses with the male pronucleus.

21. The answer is D.

Myotome cells are derived from somites and cranial somitomeres. Myotomal cells from somites form ventral and dorsal groups of migrating cells called hypomeres and epimeres, respectively. The hypomeric myotomal cells migrate into the lateral body walls of the neck, thorax, and abdomen to form the axial muscles. In the regions of the limbs, these cells also migrate into the limb buds to form the appendicular musculature. The epimeric mass of myotomal cells migrates dorsally and primarily forms the muscles of the back and posterior part of the neck. Once at these locations, the myoblasts proliferate and differentiate into myocytes. If, for some reason, the hypomeric group does not migrate, proliferate, or differentiate within the abdominal region, the abdominal musculature will not develop. Since this musculature plays a key role in supporting the abdominal wall, congenital absence of this musculature leads to a distended abdomen with wrinkled skin, commonly referred to as "prune belly."

22 and 23. The answers are A and D, respectively.

Sacrococcygeal teratomas are thought to arise from undifferentiated stem cells derived from remnants of the primitive streak. These teratomas grow quickly and, because of their primitive streak origin, differentiate into almost any cell type found in the adult body. Because the primitive streak is a caudal structure, these tumors usually develop in the sacral region. They grow rapidly and can reach sizes that sometimes complicate the delivery of the baby. The tumor tissue is usually removed as soon as possible, as between 50% and 70% of tumors become metastatic within 2 months. Teratocarcinomas are very similar but are likely derived from stray and persistent primordial germ cells. They usually form along the migratory pathway of primordial germ cells. Stray and persistent cells from molar pregnancies often form choriocarcinomas.

24. The answer is C.

DNA synthesis is required before mitosis and the first meiotic division can occur. However, there is no intervening DNA synthesis between the first and second meiotic division. Because meiosis requires 2 karyokinetic events, metaphase occurs twice. It is during the first metaphase that a major discriminating feature between meiosis and mitosis occurs. This is synapsis (pairing of homologous chromosomes). This pairing of duplicated paternal and maternal chromosomes permits crossover and also serves a centromeric function for aligning the paired chromosomes along the equatorial plate during metaphase I. During the first meiotic division, the paternal or maternal representative of each chromosome pair is segregated into separate daughter cells. Which parental chromosome each daughter cell gets is random for each chromosome pair. In contrast, during mitosis, the paternal and maternal chromosomes align separately along the metaphase equatorial plate, where the sister chromatids separate during anaphase. Consequently, each daughter cell receives an entire complement of both maternal and paternal chromatids and contains the same exact DNA complement as the parental cell.

25–27. The answers are A, C, and B, respectively.

Once puberty begins, the hypothalamus releases gonadotropin-releasing hormone every month, and in response FSH is released from the anterior pituitary. FSH stimulates the development of 5–15 primordial follicles in the ovaries. In response, the follicle cells surrounding the primary oocyte proliferate and begin synthesizing and secreting estrogen. One function of this estrogen is to drive the regrowth and regeneration of the endometrial mucosa and uterine glands. LH transforms the granulosa and thecal cells of the graafian follicle remaining after ovulation into luteal cells of the corpus luteum. Luteal cells secrete the progesterone and estrogen needed for the secretory phase of the menstrual cycle, thereby preparing the uterus for implantation.

PART II

Gastrointestinal Development I: Foregut and Stomach

A. Formation of Foregut, Midgut, and Hindgut

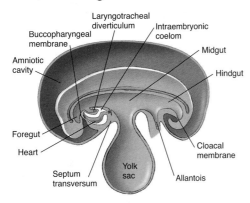

- Laryngotracheal diverticulum
- Buccopharyngeal membrane
- Intraembryonic coelom
- Amniotic cavity
- Midgut
- Hindgut
- Foregut
- Heart
- Cloacal membrane
- Septum transversum
- Yolk sac
- Allantois

B. Stomach and Mesenteries

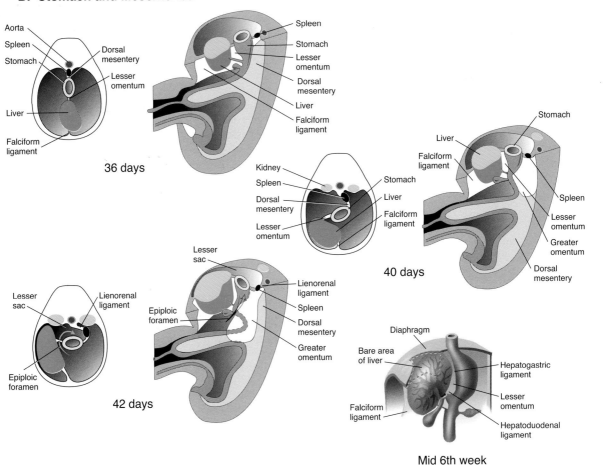

36 days
- Aorta
- Spleen
- Stomach
- Dorsal mesentery
- Lesser omentum
- Liver
- Falciform ligament

- Spleen
- Stomach
- Lesser omentum
- Dorsal mesentery
- Liver
- Falciform ligament

40 days
- Kidney
- Spleen
- Dorsal mesentery
- Lesser omentum
- Stomach
- Liver
- Falciform ligament

- Stomach
- Liver
- Falciform ligament
- Spleen
- Lesser omentum
- Greater omentum
- Dorsal mesentery

42 days
- Lesser sac
- Lienorenal ligament
- Epiploic foramen

- Lesser sac
- Lienorenal ligament
- Spleen
- Dorsal mesentery
- Greater omentum
- Epiploic foramen

Mid 6th week
- Diaphragm
- Bare area of liver
- Hepatogastric ligament
- Lesser omentum
- Falciform ligament
- Hepatoduodenal ligament

OVERVIEW

The endodermally lined yolk sac is pulled into the embryo during early body folding, forming the foregut, midgut, and hindgut. The endoderm differentiates into the epithelium and digestive glands appropriate for each segment, and the surrounding splanchnic mesoderm generates the connective tissue and smooth muscle. The foregut forms the pharynx, lower respiratory tract and esophagus, stomach, proximal duodenum, liver parenchyma, gallbladder and hepatic ducts, and pancreas. The midgut forms the remainder of the small intestine, ascending colon, and about two thirds of the transverse colon. The hindgut forms the rest.

Early Stages of Gastrointestinal (GI) Development

During the fourth week, embryonic folding pulls the endoderm of the yolk sac into the cranial and caudal ends of the embryo, forming the foregut, midgut, and hindgut (see Chapter 11). The gut tube is closed on both ends by the buccopharyngeal (cranial) and cloacal membranes (caudal) (**Part A**). Here, the endoderm and ectoderm are in direct contact with one another and are externally demarcated by shallow depressions, the stomodeum (primordial mouth) and protodeum (primordial anus). The endoderm forms the epithelial lining and associated glands of the GI tract, while the surrounding splanchnic mesoderm generates the connective tissue and smooth-muscle walls. Derivatives of the foregut include the pharynx, lower respiratory tract, esophagus, stomach, duodenum proximal to the bile duct, liver, hepatic ducts, gallbladder, and pancreas. The midgut forms the remaining small intestine, the ascending colon, and the first two thirds of the transverse colon. The hindgut forms the distal third of the transverse colon, the descending colon, sigmoid colon, rectum, and part of the anal canal. By the end of the fourth week, the gut tube caudal to the developing diaphragm is suspended from the posterior abdominal wall by a dorsal mesentery, a double fold of the peritoneum enclosing the organs (**Part B**). This mesentery extends from the lower esophagus to the caudal end of the hindgut. A ventral mesentery also develops but only in the region of the stomach. Maturation of the GI gastroepithelium is well under way by 8–10 weeks, and peristaltic contractions begin as early as week 10.

The Stomach

During the fourth week, a small portion of the foregut dilates just below the diaphragm (**Parts B** and **C**). As this dilatation enlarges to form the stomach, differential growth between its dorsal and ventral borders leads to formation of the greater and lesser curvatures of the stomach. As the stomach enlarges, it also rotates along the longitudinal body axis so that the lesser curvature moves toward the right and the dorsal curvature moves to the left. This continues until the left side of the stomach lies parallel to the ventral abdominal surface. The change in position also reorients the left and right descending vagus nerves so that they are now anterior and posterior near the level of the stomach. Concurrently, the stomach also shifts position from the midline toward the left side of abdominal cavity. The rotation of the stomach also pulls the dorsal mesentery (mesogastrium) toward the left. This mesentery lengthens, generating a double-layered fold of mesentery, called the greater omentum, that hangs from the stomach and covers the transverse colon and abdominal contents. The blind pouch between the mesentery folds is called the omental bursa, and it is obliterated by the fusion of these folds overlying the intestines. The ventral mesentery connecting the stomach to the liver becomes the lesser omentum (forming hepatoduodenal and hepatogastric ligaments). The mesentery between the developing liver and the ventral body wall forms the falciform ligament (**Parts B** and **C**). Beneath the free margin of the lesser omentum is the epiploic foramen, the opening connecting the main portion of the peritoneal cavity with the omental bursa.

Clinical Aspects

Pyloric stenosis, a narrowing of the GI tract, is caused by a thickening of the pyloric sphincter muscle wall and is relatively common (1/150 males and 1/750 females). If the stenosis is severe, it can obstruct the passage of food, distend the stomach, and cause vomiting by the infant. It requires surgical correction. Congenital hiatal hernias occur if the esophagus fails to lengthen during embryonic development, pulling the stomach superiorly through the diaphragmatic hiatus. Symptoms of these hernias usually show up in older adults because the diaphragm weakens with age and the esophageal hiatus widens.

14 Gastrointestinal Development II: Duodenum and Accesory Glands

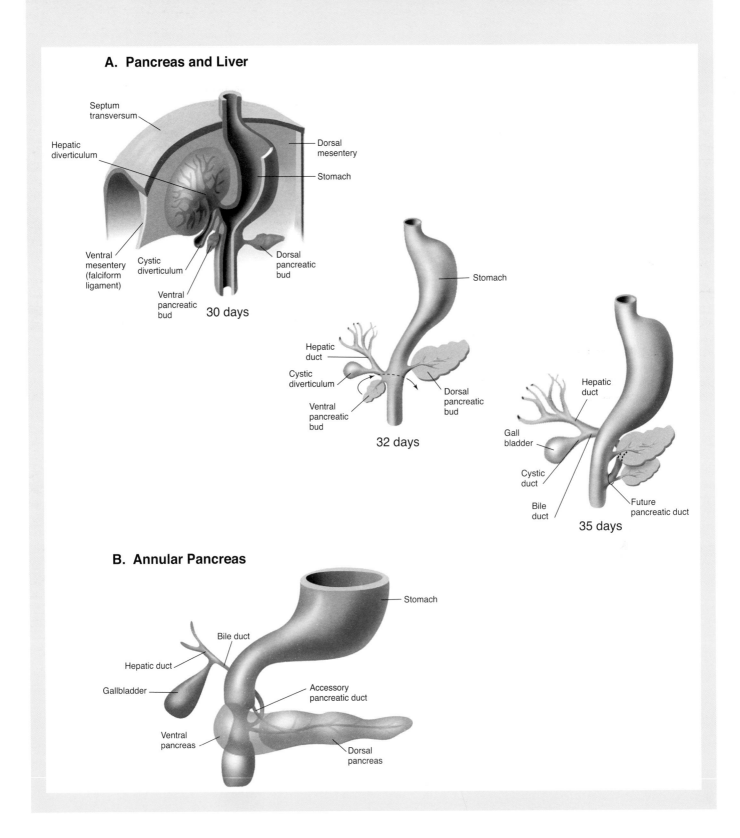

A. Pancreas and Liver

Septum transversum

Hepatic diverticulum

Dorsal mesentery

Stomach

Ventral mesentery (falciform ligament)

Cystic diverticulum

Ventral pancreatic bud

Dorsal pancreatic bud

30 days

Stomach

Hepatic duct

Cystic diverticulum

Ventral pancreatic bud

Dorsal pancreatic bud

32 days

Hepatic duct

Gall bladder

Cystic duct

Bile duct

Future pancreatic duct

35 days

B. Annular Pancreas

Stomach

Bile duct

Hepatic duct

Gallbladder

Accessory pancreatic duct

Ventral pancreas

Dorsal pancreas

OVERVIEW

The duodenum develops from both the foregut and midgut. As the stomach rotates, the duodenal segment is bent into a C-shape and becomes retroperitoneal. The lumen of the duodenum becomes temporarily obliterated as the epithelium proliferates and then recanalizes. Failure of proper recanalization leads to duodenal stenosis or atresia. The liver, gallbladder, and pancreas form from endodermal buds extending into the ventral and dorsal mesenteries. The ventral pancreatic bud rotates to the left side as the stomach and duodenum rotate, and it fuses with the dorsal pancreatic bud to make the pancreas. Acinar and ductal cells are derived from endoderm. The pancreatic islet cells are also thought to be derived from the endoderm. An annular pancreas develops when the ventral pancreatic bud wraps around both sides of the duodenum and then fuses with the dorsal bud. An annular pancreas can lead to bowel obstruction.

Duodenum

The duodenum forms from both the foregut and the midgut. As the stomach rotates, the duodenum is bent into a C-shape, becomes apposed to the abdominal wall, and becomes retroperitoneal. During the fifth and sixth weeks of development, the lumen of the duodenum becomes temporarily obliterated as the epithelial cells proliferate, and then it recanalizes by the end of the embryonic period.

Accessory Glands

The liver parenchyma, gallbladder, and associated ducts form from endodermal buds extending from the duodenal endoderm and growing into the ventral mesentery (**Part A**). Endoderm in the ventral wall of the duodenum proliferates, forming a ventral diverticulum that then branches to form a hepatic diverticulum and ventral pancreatic bud. The hepatic diverticulum continues to grow, first into the lesser omentum and then pushing into the lower part of the septum transversum. Here, the hepatic diverticulum continues to branch, forming liver cords that differentiate into hepatocytes, and hepatic ducts. Splanchnic mesoderm forms the supporting stroma, with some contribution by somatic mesoderm of the septum transversum. Meanwhile, another endodermal diverticulum, called the cystic diverticulum, forms on the hepatic diverticulum and generates the gallbladder and cystic duct.

The pancreas forms from ventral and dorsal buds originating as outgrowths of the duodenal endoderm beginning on day 26 (**Part C**). Both buds project and expand into the corresponding ventral and dorsal mesenteries. When the duodenum rotates to the right and becomes C-shaped, the ventral bud migrates dorsally and comes to lie immediately below the dorsal pancreatic bud. Eventually the pancreatic parenchyma and pancreatic ducts of the 2 heads fuse together, with the original ventral head forming the uncinate process and dorsal head forming the rest. The pancreas contains both exocrine and endocrine portions. All the acinar and ductal cells are derived from endoderm. The origin of pancreatic islet cells is unclear, but they likely originate from the endoderm. Islets develop during the third month of fetal life, and insulin secretion begins in approximately the fifth month. Glucagon-secreting and somatostatin-secreting cells also develop within the islets. Other than the nerves, the rest of the organ is derived from splanchnic mesoderm.

Clinical Aspects

Sometimes the duodenum does not recanalize. If normal recanalization does not occur, duodenal stenosis or even atresia can develop. Either can lead to hydramniotic or polyhydramniotic conditions (high level of amniotic fluid) because each prevents the normal absorption of amniotic fluid by the fetal intestines. Duodenal stenosis and atresia also cause dilatation of the cranial gut and vomiting, with the stomach contents often containing bile.

An annular pancreas develops when the ventral pancreatic bud splits and migrates around both sides of the duodenum and then fuses with the dorsal bud (**Part D**). This can constrict the duodenum, causing obstruction of the bowel. Pancreatic islet development is accelerated and fetal insulin secretion is stimulated during pregnancies of diabetic women. This can increase fetal birth weight and the risk of infant death.

15 Gastrointestinal Development III: Midgut and Hindgut

A. Rotation of Midgut and Hindgut

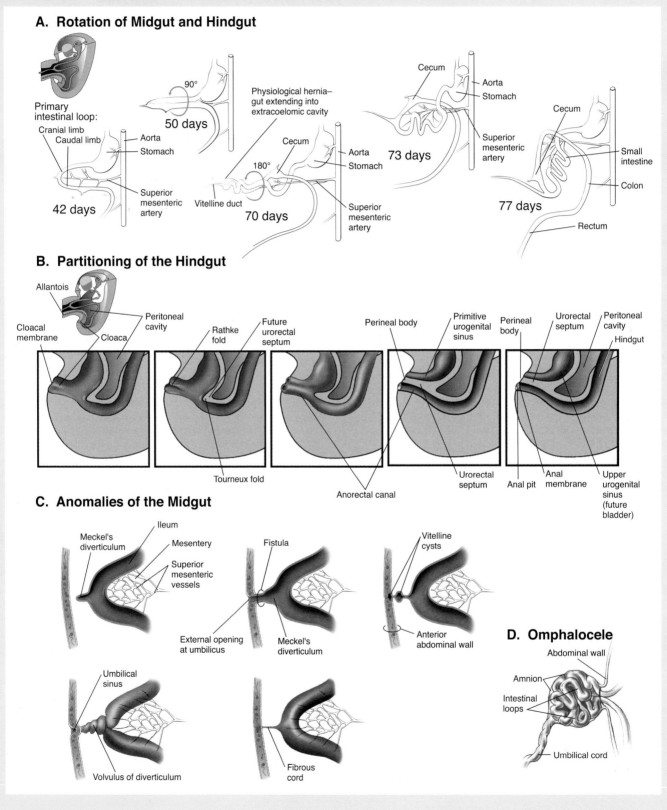

Primary intestinal loop:
Cranial limb
Caudal limb
Aorta
Stomach
Superior mesenteric artery
42 days

90°
50 days

180°
Vitelline duct
70 days
Cecum
Aorta
Stomach
Superior mesenteric artery

Physiological hernia– gut extending into extracoelomic cavity
Cecum
Aorta
Stomach
Superior mesenteric artery
73 days

Cecum
Aorta
Stomach
Superior mesenteric artery
Cecum
Small intestine
Colon
Rectum
77 days

B. Partitioning of the Hindgut

Allantois
Cloacal membrane
Cloaca
Peritoneal cavity

Rathke fold
Future urorectal septum
Tourneux fold

Perineal body
Anorectal canal

Primitive urogenital sinus
Perineal body
Urorectal septum
Anal pit
Anal membrane

Urorectal septum
Peritoneal cavity
Hindgut
Upper urogenital sinus (future bladder)

C. Anomalies of the Midgut

Meckel's diverticulum
Ileum
Mesentery
Superior mesenteric vessels

Fistula
External opening at umbilicus
Meckel's diverticulum

Vitelline cysts
Anterior abdominal wall

Umbilical sinus
Volvulus of diverticulum

Fibrous cord

D. Omphalocele

Abdominal wall
Amnion
Intestinal loops
Umbilical cord

OVERVIEW

The space required by the rapidly growing midgut exceeds the volume of the embryonic abdominal cavity. Hence, the midgut temporarily herniates into extraembryonic coelom within the umbilicus. As the midgut returns to the abdominal cavity, it begins a 270-degree counterclockwise rotation such that the cecum crosses anterior to the small intestine and ends up in the lower right abdominal cavity, with the bulk of the large intestine forming an inverted U-shaped loop. The hindgut forms not only the remainder of the large intestine and rectum but also part of the urinary system. Separation of the anorectal portion of the hindgut from the urinary portion requires formation of the urorectal septum. Abnormal partitioning of the hindgut can lead to several different types of congenital anomalies.

Physiological Umbilical Herniation of the Midgut

By the fifth week, the midgut is suspended from the abdominal wall by the dorsal mesentery and is continuous with the yolk sac via the vitelline duct (yolk stalk). At this site, the intraembryonic coelom (in this case the abdominal cavity) is continuous with the extraembryonic coelom found within the primitive umbilical cord. As the midgut rapidly increases in length, it forms a U-shaped loop that projects into the extraembryonic coelom, as the abdominal cavity is too small to accommodate the rapidly growing midgut (**Part A**). This physiological umbilical hernia (a normal, nonpathological hernia) begins forming during the sixth week.

Rotation of Midgut

The segment of the midgut superior to the vitelline duct is referred to as the *cranial limb,* while the segment inferior to it is called the *caudal limb* (**Part A**). The cranial limb undergoes the greatest elongation and forms the small intestine, while the caudal limb develops into the ascending and transverse colon. As the midgut loop herniates into the umbilicus, it begins rotating in a 90-degree counterclockwise direction (as viewed from the front) around the long axis of the herniated loop. Therefore, the cranial limb is now located on the right and the caudal limb is on the left. As the superior limb lengthens and differentiates into the jejunum and ileum, the dorsal mesentery is thrown into folds. Meanwhile, the caudal limb forms the cecum and a diverticulum called the *appendix.* By the 10th week, the midgut begins retracting back into the abdomen, while the intestines rotate an additional 180 degrees. During this rotation, the cecum moves cranially and toward the right, passing in front of the small intestine. The cecum then descends, ending up in the lower right abdominal cavity and causing the remaining caudal limb to take on an inverted U-shaped configuration. The dorsal mesenteries of the ascending and descending segments of the future colon then shorten, pulling these segments up against the abdominal wall where they become retroperitoneal. By the beginning of the 11th week, the entire midgut is back within the abdominal cavity, and the connection between the yolk sac and midgut is eventually obliterated.

The Hindgut

The hindgut forms a part of the transverse colon and the entire descending and sigmoid colon. The hindgut also forms the rectum and anus through a complex process. Early in development, the terminal hindgut dilates, forming the cloaca and a slender superior-ventral diverticulum called the *allantois* (**Part B**). Separating the cloaca from the exterior is the ectoderm and endoderm of the cloacal membrane. The cloaca is partitioned into the rectum and the urogenital sinus (terminal part of the urinary system) by formation of a urorectal (urogenital) septum. This septum is thought to form from a wedge of mesoderm that develops between the anterior and posterior portions of the cloaca. This wedge extends caudally and fuses with 2 lateral mesodermal folds growing toward the midline from either side of the cloaca (Rathke folds). Eventually the urorectal septum fuses with the cloacal membrane marking the site of the perineal body, dividing the posterior-most compartment of the cloaca (the anorectal canal) from the more anterior compartment (the urogenital sinus). The superior two thirds of the adult anorectal canal is derived from the hindgut, but the lower third is derived from an ectoderm pit called the *anal pit.* This pit forms because of mesodermal proliferation surrounding the cloacal membrane. Eventually, the cloacal membrane in this region ruptures during the eighth week, the rupture site being demarcated by the pectinate line within the anorectal canal. Failure to rupture leads to anal atresia (1/5,000 incidence).

Clinical Aspects

A small portion of the vitelline duct within the abdomen sometimes persists, forming an outpocketing of ileum of varying length in 2%–4% of the population. This outpocketing is called *Meckel's diverticulum* (**Part C**). While it may be asymptomatic, it can lead to bowel obstructions. The wall of the diverticulum contains the same layers as the ileum, but the mucosa also may contain patches of pancreatic or gastric mucosa. Sometimes the vitelline duct persists and remains patent, forming an open connection between the ileum and exterior abdominal surface. This is called an *omphalomesenteric* or *umbilical fistula.* The vitelline duct also may persist as a fibrous cord connecting the ileum with the umbilicus, and occasionally the cord may contain intervening vitelline cysts (enterocysts). The presence of this cord greatly increases the risk of developing a volvulus (intestinal twisting), leading to intestinal obstruction, bowel septis, or GI bleeding. If the intestines fail to re-enter the abdominal cavity, they protrude into the coelom of the umbilicus and are covered by the epithelium of the umbilical cord. This is called an *omphalocele* (1/5,000 incidence), and almost 25% of affected fetuses die before birth (**Part D**). Those that survive require immediate surgical repair. Omphalocele is different from gastroschisis, in which the defect occurs as a consequence of failed closure of the ventral abdominal wall. In gastroschisis, the abdominal contents protrude directly out of the abdominal cavity and are in direct contact with amniotic fluid or in the case of a newborn, the air. Nonrotation of the gut (*left-sided colon*), is generally asymptomatic but may be accompanied by volvulus. Sometimes the gut rotates in the opposite direction, reversing the sidedness of the organs but retaining their proper orientation with respect to one another.

Rectal atresia is a congenital anomaly whereby the anus and rectum remain separated from one another. It is likely caused by defects in formation of the urorectal septum or by abnormal recanalization of the colon. Rectal atresia is often accompanied by fistulas that can connect the rectum to the outer perineum or to the urogenital system, depending on whether the rectum ends superiorly or inferiorly to the puborectalis muscle. Several possible fistulas, including rectovaginal, rectourethral, rectoprostatic, and rectouterine fistulas, can develop.

16 | Urogenital System I: The Kidney

A. Primitive Kidneys

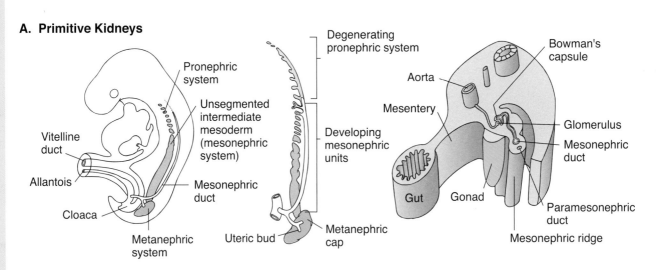

B. Metanephric Kidneys

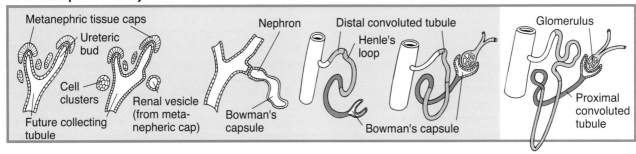

C. Ascent of Kidneys

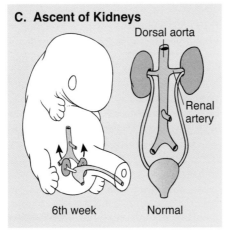

D. Abnormal Kidney

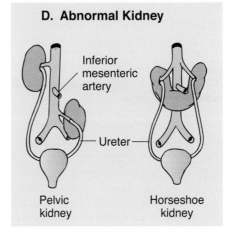

OVERVIEW

Intermediate mesoderm generates the entire kidney. Two transient primitive kidneys form and regress before the permanent metanephric kidney develops. Metanephric kidney development begins with the formation of a sprouting ureteric bud covered by a cap of condensed intermediate (metanephric cap) mesoderm. The ureteric bud elongates and branches, eventually forming the collecting tubules, major and minor calyces, renal pelvis, and ureters. The metanephric caps develop short tubules that make Bowman's capsule, the proximal and distal convoluted tubules, and the loops of Henle. The renal vessels and glomerular capillaries form from adjacent mesoderm.

Origins of the Early Urogenital System

The urogenital system is generally divided into 2 different components, the urinary system and the genital system. These 2 systems develop in conjunction with one another and are almost entirely derived from intermediate mesoderm. The intermediate mesoderm usually remains associated with the posterior body cavity, but near the caudal end of the embryo, it grows and fuses with the ventrolateral walls of the cloacal mesoderm.

Early Excretory Units

Beginning in the fourth week, the intermediate mesoderm forms a longitudinal ridge called the *urogenital ridge* that protrudes into the coelomic cavity. Within each ridge, 3 different overlapping segmental kidney systems progressively develop. They are the pronephros, mesonephros, and metanephros kidneys (**Part A**). The pronephros kidney forms in the cervical region, generating rudimentary excretory tubules that never function. The pronephros kidney regresses as the more caudal mesonephric kidney develops within the thoracic and upper lumbar regions. In the mesonephric region, some of the mesoderm forms S-shaped tubules that expand on their medial end, making Bowman's capsule, while adjacent mesoderm forms glomeruli (collectively making a primitive renal corpuscle) (**Part A**). Laterally, these tubules open into a longitudinal tube forming within the urogenital ridge, called the *mesonephric duct* (wolffian duct). This duct serves as a primitive collecting duct and opens into the cloaca. The mesonephric kidney becomes functional between the 6th and 10th weeks, dumping small amounts of urine into the mesonephric duct and cloaca. Meanwhile, the renal mesoderm condenses to form a large ovoid organ on either side of the midline. By the end of the second month, however, the cranial-most mesonephric tubules and much of the mesonephric duct begin to degenerate (in males much of the mesonephric duct is retained; see Chapter 18).

Metanephric Kidney

As the mesonephric kidney degenerates, the metanephric kidney (permanent kidney) begins to develop. At the caudal end of each mesonephric duct, a sprout called a *ureteric bud* begins to form (**Part A**). This bud induces the adjacent intermediate mesoderm to form a cluster of cells called the *metanephric mesodermal cap.*

Tissue–tissue Interactions between the bud and cap induce continued branching and elongation of the ureteric bud and continued proliferation of the metanephric cap mesoderm. Eventually, the ureteric buds differentiate and form the ureters, the renal calyces, and the renal pelvis of the adult kidney, with the final divisions of the branching ureteric buds forming the collecting ducts and tubules (**Part B**). The metanephric mesodermal caps eventually form Bowman's capsule, the proximal convoluted tubule, the loops of Henle, and the distal convoluted tubule. The distal convoluted tubule eventually opens into the collecting tubule. Glomerular capillaries form from adjacent mesoderm and eventually connect to the dorsal aorta.

Formation of these nephrons continues throughout fetal life with at least 15 generations of branching, each getting closer to the cortex of the organ. Because of this branching, the fetal and newborn kidney has a lobulated appearance, but this eventually disappears as the nephrons grow. While initially located in the pelvis, the metanephric kidney moves cranially as the lumbar and sacral body regions grow and the mesonephric kidney regresses (**Part C**).

Clinical Aspects

Occasionally, a kidney fails to ascend and remains in the pelvis (pelvic kidney) (**Part D**). Sometimes the caudal portions of the 2 metanephric kidneys fuse with one another over the ventral surface of the aorta, forming a horseshoe-shaped kidney (1/600 incidence). When this happens, the fused kidneys become trapped beneath the inferior mesenteric artery.

Congenital polycystic kidney is a condition whereby numerous cysts form within the kidney, resulting in renal insufficiency and eventual kidney failure. This condition may be inherited as an autosomal recessive or dominant trait or result from an unknown etiology. It appears to stem from abnormal development or function of the proximal convoluted tube, collecting system, or ureteric bud. Occasionally, one or both kidneys may not develop at all, resulting in unilateral (1/1,000 incidence) or bilateral (1/3,000 incidence) renal agenesis. This condition may result from a degeneration of the ureteric bud with subsequent loss of the metanephric cap. Bilateral renal agenesis usually leads to an oligohydramniotic condition (insufficient amniotic fluid) because without functioning kidneys, the fetus cannot excrete into the amniotic fluid.

17 Urogenital System II: Bladder and Urethra

A. Partitioning of the Hindgut

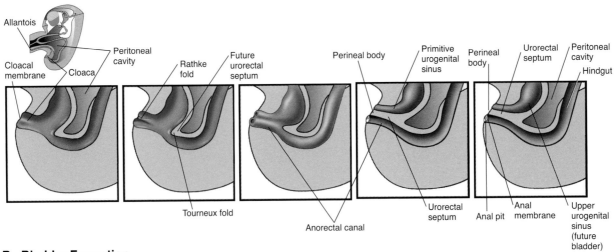

Allantois

Cloacal membrane

Cloaca

Peritoneal cavity

Rathke fold

Future urorectal septum

Tourneux fold

Anorectal canal

Perineal body

Primitive urogenital sinus

Urorectal septum

Perineal body

Urorectal septum

Peritoneal cavity

Hindgut

Anal pit

Anal membrane

Upper urogenital sinus (future bladder)

B. Bladder Formation

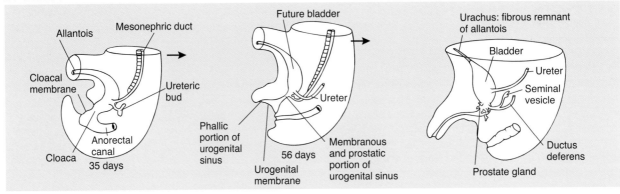

Allantois

Mesonephric duct

Cloacal membrane

Ureteric bud

Anorectal canal

Cloaca

35 days

Future bladder

Phallic portion of urogenital sinus

Urogenital membrane

56 days

Ureter

Membranous and prostatic portion of urogenital sinus

Urachus: fibrous remnant of allantois

Bladder

Ureter

Seminal vesicle

Ductus deferens

Prostate gland

C. Anomalies

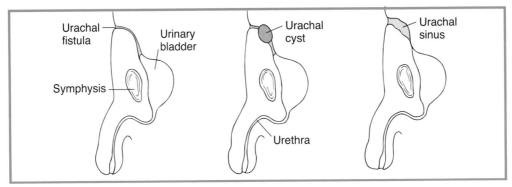

Urachal fistula

Urinary bladder

Symphysis

Urachal cyst

Urethra

Urachal sinus

OVERVIEW

The urorectal (urogenital) septum separates the cloaca into two compartments, the anorectal canal and the urogenital sinus. The urogenital sinus is further subdivided into a larger upper portion that forms the bladder and a smaller lower portion that forms the urethra. The developing ureters empty into the portion forming the bladder. The urogenital sinus is also continuous with the allantois. The allantois extends from the developing bladder into the umbilical cord. It is eventually obliterated, forming the urachus. Several anomalies result from improper development of the urorectal septum and urogenital sinus.

Bladder and Urethra Formation

As discussed in Chapter 15, the developing urorectal septum separates the endodermally lined cloaca into 2 compartments, the anorectal canal (future anus and rectum) and the urogenital sinus (future bladder and urethra). The upper and largest portion of the urogenital sinus forms the bladder (**Parts A** and **B**). As the bladder wall expands, it incorporates the caudal portion of the mesonephric duct and engulfs the roots of the ureteric buds so that eventually the ureters open directly into the dorsal surface of the bladder. In males, the mesonephric ducts are retained. As the bladder wall expands and the kidneys ascend, the mesonephric ducts are carried toward the midline via differential growth. The mesonephric ducts eventually empty into the lower urogenital sinus at the site of the future prostatic urethra, where they will form the vas deferens, seminal vesicles, and ejaculatory ducts.

The developing bladder is also continuous with the allantois. The allantois extends into the umbilicus and is eventually obliterated as the umbilicus closes. The fibrous remnant of the allantois within the abdominal cavity is recognized in the adult as the urachus and runs between the apex of the bladder and the umbilicus. In the adult, the peritoneum overlies the urachus, and together they form a ligament called the *median umbilical ligament*.

The lower portion of the urogenital sinus narrows and forms the membranous urethra in females and both the membranous and prostatic uretheras in males. Here, epithelial buds develop and grow into the surrounding splanchnic mesoderm, where they form the paraurethral glands in females and prostate gland in males. Finally, the last portion of the urogenital sinus is the phallic portion. In this region, the urogenital sinus extends anteriorly a short distance while still remaining superior to the cloacal membrane. The development of this portion of the urethra differs between the sexes (see Chapters 18 and 19). During these early stages, the urogenital sinus compartment is still separated from the outer surface by the cloacal membrane, but eventually this membrane ruptures.

Clinical Aspects

A urachal fistula occurs when the lumen of the abdominal portion of the allantois persists, and urine may be observed draining from the umbilicus (**Part C**). If only a small area of the allantois remains, a urachal cyst forms, and if the distal portion of the allantois remains open, a urachal sinus forms. Exstrophy of the bladder (1/50,000 incidence) is a rare congenital defect in which the ventral wall of the bladder is open and the bladder mucosa is exposed to the outside environment. It is usually accompanied by an open urinary tract running from the phallus to the umbilicus. It may be caused by a deficit in mesodermal cell migration and proliferation in this region. As discussed in Chapter 15, incomplete separation of the urogenital sinus from the anorectal canal or improper development of the anus often leads to formation of fistulas, including rectourethral and rectovesicular fistulas.

18 Urogenital System III: Male Reproductive System

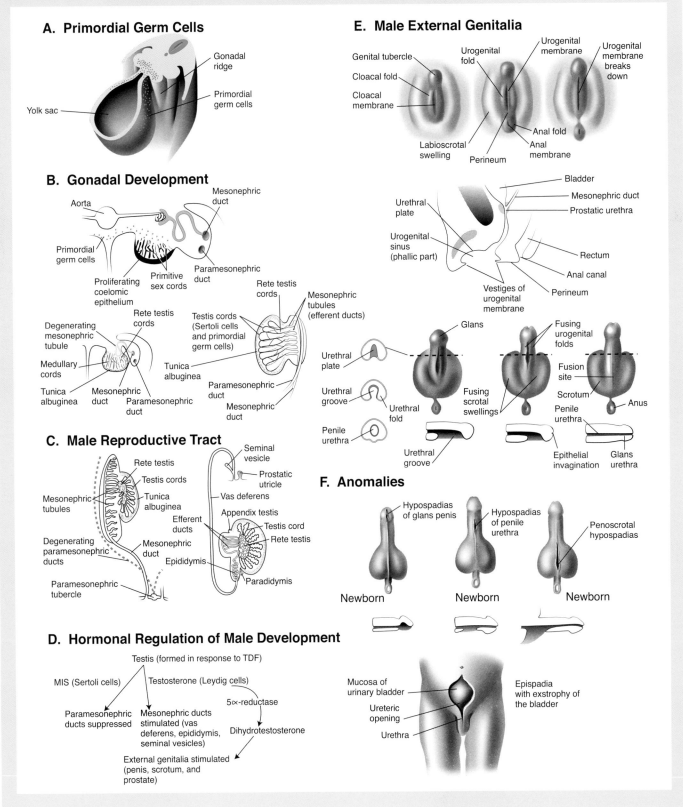

A. Primordial Germ Cells

Gonadal ridge
Primordial germ cells
Yolk sac

B. Gonadal Development

Aorta
Mesonephric duct
Primordial germ cells
Paramesonephric duct
Proliferating coelomic epithelium
Primitive sex cords
Rete testis cords
Mesonephric tubules (efferent ducts)
Degenerating mesonephric tubule
Rete testis cords
Testis cords (Sertoli cells and primordial germ cells)
Medullary cords
Tunica albuginea
Tunica albuginea
Mesonephric duct
Paramesonephric duct
Paramesonephric duct
Mesonephric duct

C. Male Reproductive Tract

Seminal vesicle
Rete testis
Prostatic utricle
Testis cords
Vas deferens
Tunica albuginea
Appendix testis
Mesonephric tubules
Efferent ducts
Testis cord
Rete testis
Degenerating paramesonephric ducts
Mesonephric duct
Epididymis
Paradidymis
Paramesonephric tubercle

D. Hormonal Regulation of Male Development

Testis (formed in response to TDF)
MIS (Sertoli cells)
Testosterone (Leydig cells)
5∝-reductase
Paramesonephric ducts suppressed
Mesonephric ducts stimulated (vas deferens, epididymis, seminal vesicles)
Dihydrotestosterone
External genitalia stimulated (penis, scrotum, and prostate)

E. Male External Genitalia

Genital tubercle
Urogenital fold
Urogenital membrane
Urogenital membrane breaks down
Cloacal fold
Cloacal membrane
Labioscrotal swelling
Perineum
Anal fold
Anal membrane

Bladder
Urethral plate
Mesonephric duct
Prostatic urethra
Urogenital sinus (phallic part)
Rectum
Anal canal
Vestiges of urogenital membrane
Perineum

Glans
Fusing urogenital folds
Urethral plate
Fusion site
Urethral groove
Fusing scrotal swellings
Urethral fold
Scrotum
Penile urethra
Anus
Penile urethra
Urethral groove
Epithelial invagination
Glans urethra

F. Anomalies

Hypospadias of glans penis
Hypospadias of penile urethra
Penoscrotal hypospadias
Newborn
Newborn
Newborn

Mucosa of urinary bladder
Ureteric opening
Urethra
Epispadia with exstrophy of the bladder

OVERVIEW

The development of the male and female reproductive systems is very similar. Reproductive development begins with the formation of the gonadal ridge within the intermediate mesoderm. This ridge is populated by primordial germ cells originating in the yolk sac wall that in turn stimulate the gonadal ridge epithelium to form either Sertoli cells or follicular cells. Whether the gonad becomes a testis or ovary depends on the Y chromosome. Without this chromosome, the gonad becomes an ovary. Growth factors and hormones produced by the specific gonadal type direct the subsequent development of mesonephric and paramesonephric ducts and external genitalia toward gender-specific forms.

Indifferent Gonads

The formation of a particular gonad type involves both autosomes and sex chromosomes, but the key to sexual dimorphism is the Y chromosome. This chromosome encodes testis-determining factor (TDF), the presence or absence of which directs gonadal differentiation. All embryos without the Y chromosome develop as females. The primitive gonads initially appear as a pair of longitudinal ridges forming within the intermediate mesoderm adjacent to the mesonephric kidneys. Primordial germ cells differentiate within the yolk sac mesoderm near the hindgut and migrate into the gonadal ridges by the sixth week (**Part A**). Without these cells, the gonads do not develop. Once there, the primordial germ cells stimulate the overlying coelomic epithelium to proliferate and penetrate the underlying mesenchyme, forming irregular cords of cells called *primitive sex cords* (**Part B**).

Development of the Testis

In the presence of TDF, the primitive sex cords lose contact with the surface and form medullary cords. Eventually, these cells differentiate into Sertoli cells, surround the primordial germ cells, and organize into U-shaped loops that form the definitive seminiferous tubules at puberty. Unlike their female counterparts, male primordial germ cells do not differentiate into spermatogonia until puberty. The medullary cord cells farthest away from the gonadal surface form the rete testis and connect the future seminiferous tubules with the efferent ductules. The Leydig cells differentiate from the mesoderm lying between the cords and by the 9th–10th week begin producing testosterone.

Male Reproductive Tract

As discussed in Chapter 16, the mesonephric duct (wolffian duct) serves as a collecting duct for the mesonephric kidney and runs in close proximity to the genital ridge. Another duct forms by an evagination of the urogenital ridge epithelium running parallel to each mesonephric duct. This duct, the paramesonephric duct (müllerian duct), opens into the coelomic cavity at its cranial end and fuses with the corresponding contralateral paramesonephric duct at the caudal end before reaching the urogenital sinus. Retention and remodeling of both duct systems into gender-specific reproductive organs are dependent on the type of gonad that develops (**Parts C** and **D**). Sertoli cells produce a substance known as müllerian-inhibiting substance (MIS) that causes the paramesonephric ducts to regress. In mature males, remnants of the paramesonephric duct are represented by the appendix of the testis (the vesicular appendage attached to the upper pole of the testis) and prostatic utricle (a small structure in the prostatic urethra homologous to the upper vagina) (**Part C**). In contrast, the mesonephric duct is retained and forms the efferent ductules, epididymis, seminal vesicles, vas deferens, and ejaculatory ducts under the influence of testosterone. Testosterone produced by the Leydig cells is converted to dihydrotestosterone by the enzyme 5α-reductase, and this androgen is primarily responsible for mediating the differentiation of male external genitalia (see below).

Male External Genitalia

Beginning in the third week, the mesoderm underlying the ectoderm on both sides of the cloacal membrane forms 2 swellings called *cloacal folds* (**Part E**). At the ventral end, these cloacal folds fuse in midline to form the genital tubercle. After separation of the cloaca into urogenital and anorectal sinuses, the folds surrounding the urogenital sinus are specifically referred to as *urethral* or *urogenital folds*. The cloacal membrane is also separated into a urogenital and anal membrane. An additional pair of folds, called *labioscrotal (genital) swellings,* form lateral to the urethral folds. Soon the urogenital membrane ruptures, opening the phallic portion of the urogenital sinus to the exterior. At this point, the external genitalia of males and females are indistinguishable from one another.

The formation of male external genitalia is dependent on the androgens (e.g., dihydrotestosterone) synthesized and secreted by the fetal testis. In the presence of male steroids, the genital tubercle elongates to form the phallus and carries with it the urethral folds and a narrow extension of the endodermally lined urogenital sinus called the *urethral plate* (**Part E**). The urethral plate develops a groove extending almost the entire length of the phallus. By the end of the first trimester, the urethral folds on both sides of the urethral groove fuse in the midline, forming the penile urethra. At the distal end of the penis, a cord of ectoderm grows into the glans, fuses with the developing penile urethra, and canalizes to form the external urethral meatus. Meanwhile, the labioscrotal swellings enlarge and fuse with one another to form the scrotum.

Clinical Aspects

In males, hypospadias (1/300 incidence) results when the urethral folds fail to fuse or fusion is incomplete (**Part F**); consequently, the urethra opens on the inferior (ventral) aspect of the penis. Occasionally, it may be open along the entire length of the penis and scrotum. In epispadias (1/30,000 incidence), the urethral meatus opens dorsal to the penis. Here, the genital tubercle forms at the urorectal septum rather than at the cranial end of the urogenital sinus. Consequently, the urethral plate is cranial to the genital tubercle, and the bladder outlet is found on the dorsal side of the penis (**Part F**). Anomalies related to hermaphrodism and pseudohermaphrodism are discussed in Chapter 20.

A. Primordial Cells

B. Gonadal Development

C. Female Reproductive Tract

D. Hormonal Regulation of Female Development

Ovary (formed in absence of TDF)
 no Sertoli cells then no MIS
 no Leydig cells then no testosterone
Estrogen (maternal and placenta)

Paramesonephric ducts
stimulated (uterine tube, uterus,
upper part of vagina)

External genitalia
stimulated (labia, clitoris
lower part of vagina)

E. Uterine and Vaginal Development

F. Female External Genitalia

G. Anomalies of the Uterus and Vagina

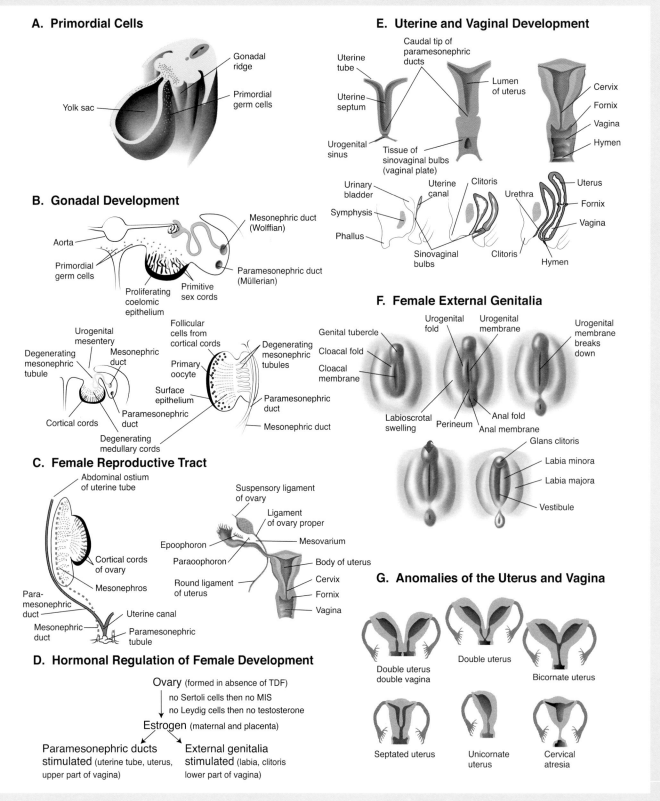

OVERVIEW

The development of the male and female reproductive systems is very similar. Development of the female reproductive system begins with the formation of gonadal ridges within the intermediate mesoderm. These ridges are populated by primordial germ cells originating in the yolk sac wall. In the absence of the Y chromosome, these germ cells differentiate into oogonia and stimulate the gonadal ridge epithelium to form follicular cells that together with other mesenchyme form the ovaries. Growth factors and hormones produced by the ovaries direct the subsequent development of the paramesonephric duct into the oviducts, uterus, and part of the vagina, while the mesonephric duct system regresses. Estrogen, primarily derived from maternal and placental sources, drives the formation of external genitalia toward a female gender-specific type.

Ovarian Development

The primitive gonads initially appear as a pair of longitudinal ridges forming within the intermediate mesoderm adjacent to the mesonephric kidneys. Primordial germ cells differentiate within the yolk sac mesoderm and migrate into the gonadal ridges by the sixth week (**Part A**). Once there, the primordial germ cells stimulate the overlying coelomic epithelium to proliferate and penetrate the underlying mesenchyme, forming irregular cords of cells called *primitive sex cords* (**Part B**). In the absence of a Y chromosome, the primitive sex cords (also called medullary cords) degenerate, but a second wave of cord formation begins. These secondary cords remain near the surface and are called *cortical cords*. The primordial germ cells proliferate and differentiate into oogonia. As the oogonia proliferate, cells of the cortical cords surround the oogonia and differentiate into follicle cells. Together they form the primordial follicles. The oogonia then differentiate into primary oocytes and begin meiosis, but meiosis is halted by interactions with the follicle cells and the oocytes remain in this state until puberty. No oogonia remain postnatally, and many of the oocytes degenerate before birth.

Female Reproductive Ducts

Just as in the male, development of the female duct system depends on the type of gonad formed in the embryo (**Parts C** and **D**). Two independent duct systems develop within the urogenital ridge in males and females, the mesonephric and paramesonephric ducts. In males, the developing Sertoli cells produce MIS, which causes the paramesonephric ducts to regress. But in female embryos, the paramesonephric ducts are retained because follicle cells develop rather than MIS-producing Sertoli cells. During the embryonic and fetal period, these paramesonephric ducts develop into the oviducts (unfused portion), the uterus, and the upper third of the vagina (**Parts C** and **E**). In the absence of Leydig cells, testosterone levels are insufficient to retain the mesonephric ducts, and they regress, although some vestiges remain. These vestiges include the epoophoron and paroophoron found within the broad ligament. Some remnants of the mesonephric ducts near the uterus or upper vagina can form cysts called *Gartner's cysts*.

The upper portion of the vagina is formed from the lower segment of the fused paramesonephric ducts (**Part E**). The lower portion is derived from the vaginal (sinovaginal) plate, a thickened area of the urogenital sinus endoderm that forms adjacent to the fused paramesonephric ducts. The endoderm of the vaginal plate proliferates and forms a solid rod that then canalizes and opens into the paramesonephric lumen. However, the lumen of the vagina remains separated from the urogenital sinus by a thin membrane called the *hymen*. The hymen usually develops a small opening at some time during perinatal life. Differential growth and remodeling reposition the vagina posterior to the urethra.

Female External Genitalia

Development of the external genitalia depends on the circulating levels of androgens. In female embryos and fetuses, maternal and placental estrogens mask the low levels of masculinizing androgens. In the absence of the testosterone-producing Leydig cells of the testes, the genital tubercle forms a much smaller structure called the *clitoris* (**Part F**). In addition, the urethral folds and labioscrotal swellings found on either side of the endodermally lined urethral plate do not fuse in the midline as they do in the male. Instead, they develop into the labia minora and labia majora, with the intervening urogenital groove forming the vestibule.

Clinical Aspects

Several anomalies related to development of the uterus and vagina can occur. Many are attributable to abnormal fusion or regression of the caudal portion of the paramesonephric ducts (**Part G**). Incomplete fusion of the lower segments of the paramesonephric ducts leads to the development of a duplicated uterus with or without a duplicated vagina, a bicornate uterus (2 uterine bodies with a single cervical portion), a septated uterus, a unicornate uterus, or atresia of the cervix. Congenital absence of the vagina (1/4,000–5,000 female births) results if the vaginal plate does not form. In addition, the entire uterus may be missing, as tissue-tissue interactions responsible for inducing the vaginal plate are thought to originate from the paramesonephric ducts. The developing ureters open into the urogenital sinus, but because of their close proximity to the vaginal plate, the ureters may sometimes open ectopically into the vagina. Anomalies of the female external genitalia primarily result from abnormal hormone levels. Increased levels of certain androgens can masculinize the genital swellings, leading to an enlargement of the clitoris and scrotalization of the labioscrotal swellings. Anomalies related to hermaphrodism and pseudohermaphrodism are discussed in Chapter 20. Several anomalies also can result from abnormal partitioning of the cloaca. These include various fistulas between the rectum, bladder, and vagina.

20 Urogenital System V: Gonadal Descent and Abnormal Genital Development

A. Mesenteries of the Gonads

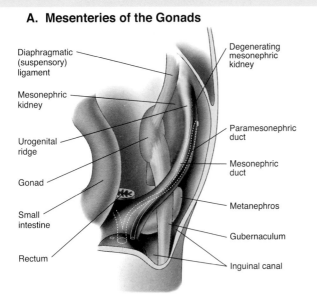

- Diaphragmatic (suspensory) ligament
- Mesonephric kidney
- Urogenital ridge
- Gonad
- Small intestine
- Rectum
- Degenerating mesonephric kidney
- Paramesonephric duct
- Mesonephric duct
- Metanephros
- Gubernaculum
- Inguinal canal

C. Anomalies of the Inguinal Canal

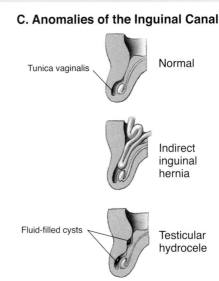

- Tunica vaginalis — Normal
- Indirect inguinal hernia
- Fluid-filled cysts — Testicular hydrocele

B. Descent of the Testes and the Inguinal Canal

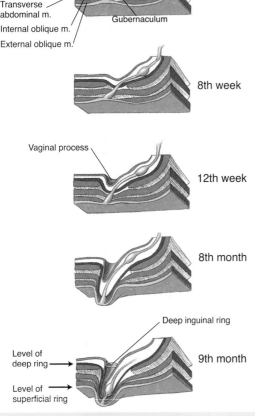

- Peritoneum
- Subserous fascia
- Transverse fascia
- Transverse abdominal m.
- Internal oblique m.
- External oblique m.
- Gubernaculum
- 7th week
- 8th week
- Vaginal process
- 12th week
- 8th month
- Deep inguinal ring
- Level of deep ring
- Level of superficial ring
- 9th month

D. Descent of the Ovaries

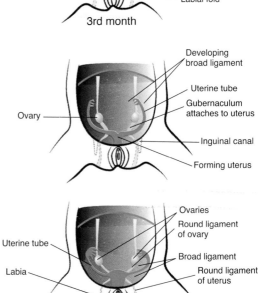

- Diaphragm
- Ovary
- Gubernaculum
- Diaphragmatic (suspensory) ligament
- Peritoneal fold (future broad ligament)
- Labial fold
- 3rd month
- Developing broad ligament
- Uterine tube
- Gubernaculum attaches to uterus
- Inguinal canal
- Forming uterus
- Ovary
- Ovaries
- Round ligament of ovary
- Broad ligament
- Round ligament of uterus
- Uterine tube
- Labia
- 7th month

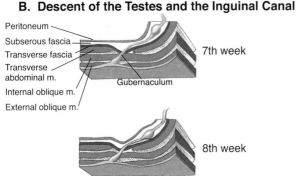
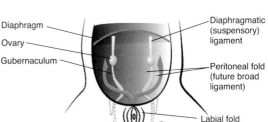

OVERVIEW

Both male and female gonads descend but do so to a much greater extent in males. A protrusion of the peritoneum through the abdominal wall into the labioscrotal swellings forms the inguinal canal and, in males, the spermatic cord. In females, the gonads remain within the abdomen but are suspended within the mesentery. Congenital anomalies occur as a consequence of abnormal hormone levels or hormone insensitivity during the embryonic and fetal period, particularly anomalies concerning the external genitalia. In cases of pseudohermaphrodism, individuals develop external genitalia mimicking sexual characteristics opposite to their genotypic and gonadal sex.

Mesenteries of the Gonads

The testes and ovaries develop near the 10th thoracic vertebral level, and both descend during embryonic and fetal life. The gonads are connected to the posterior abdominal wall, but this connection is reduced to just a simple mesentery as the mesonephric kidney regresses. Cranially, the gonadal mesentery extends toward the diaphragm along the posterior abdominal wall (**Part A**). Caudally, the mesentery extends from the gonad to the abdominal fascia adjacent to the developing labioscrotal swellings. This caudal mesentery thickens to form the gubernaculum. At the same time, an outpocketing of peritoneum forms and projects into the labioscrotal swellings adjacent to the gubernaculum. This pocket, called the *vaginal process,* pushes into the labioscrotal swellings, forming a canal called the *inguinal canal* (**Part B**). A sheath composed of successive layers of the outer abdominal wall covers this canal. The opening of the inguinal canal within the transverse fascia is the deep inguinal ring, and the external opening within the external abdominal oblique aponeurosis is the superficial inguinal ring.

Descent of the Testis

In males, the testes are carried through the inguinal canal and into the developing scrotum as the gubernaculum shortens (**Part B**). The vas deferens, testicular artery and veins, and nerves are dragged along with the testis and, together with the outer sheath, make up the spermatic cord. The innermost layer of the spermatic cord is derived from the transverse fascia and forms the internal spermatic fascia. Outside this layer, the internal abdominal oblique layer forms the cremasteric fascia and muscle, and outside this, the external abdominal oblique layer forms the external spermatic fascia. The transverse abdominal muscle layer does not contribute to the spermatic cord because it arches superiorly over the region where the vaginal process protrudes. Once the testes are in the scrotum, the vaginal process is obliterated except within the scrotum, where it becomes the tunica vaginalis. The testes eventually bulge into the tunica vaginalis. Occasionally, a communication between the tunica vaginalis and the abdomen persists, thereby increasing the likelihood of an indirect inguinal hernia (**Part C**). Sometimes, portions of the vaginal process above the testes form cysts that may fill with fluid and enlarge, forming a hydrocele of the testis or spermatic cord.

What drives the descent of the testes is unclear, but it is very dependent on the androgens produced by the fetus. Testicular descent is usually well under way by the 26th week, and by birth the testes are usually found within the scrotum. However, the arrival time varies greatly between individuals and can differ between the 2 testes in a single individual. In full-term males, 3%–4% have their testes located within the abdomen or inguinal canal. This condition, called *cryptorchism,* often rectifies itself within a year. Cryptorchid testes generate spermatozoa but usually cannot undergo spermiogenesis. Individuals with cryptorchid testes also run a 50% greater risk of developing testicular malignancies.

Descent of Ovaries

The ovaries also are anchored to the labioscrotal swellings via a gubernaculum. However, each gubernaculum becomes attached to the fusing paramesonephric ducts (future uterus) (**Part D**). Consequently, the ovaries are pulled into the abdominal cavity but descend only as far as the pelvic rim. As the gubernaculum is pulled toward the midline by the forming uterus, peritoneal folds develop over each gubernaculum and fuse together, forming the broad ligament of the ovary and the uterus. The portion of the gubernaculum between the ovary and the uterus becomes the round ligament of the ovary. The portion between the uterus and labioscrotal swellings forms the round ligament of the uterus and exits the abdomen through the deep inguinal ring, terminating within the labia major. The mesentery cranial to the ovary containing the ovarian vessels and nerves becomes the suspensory ligament of the ovary.

Clinical Aspects

Several anomalies occur as a consequence of abnormal sexual differentiation of the gonads or abnormal hormone levels. True hermaphrodites have both testicular and ovarian tissue. These individuals usually have a uterus and external genitalia that are either ambiguous or predominantly female. True hermaphrodism is extremely rare.

More common are pseudohermaphrodites, in whom the genotypic sex is masked by a phenotypic appearance closely resembling that of the opposite sex. In male pseudohermaphrodism (46, XY), the individual has testes but exhibits female-like external genitalia. There can be several causes. There may be an inadequate production of male steroids, possibly because of deficiencies in steroidal synthetic enzymes. For example, 5α-reductase deficiency decreases dihydrotestosterone levels, and consequently the development of male external genitalia is impeded. Genotypic males with androgen insensitivity syndrome (testicular feminization syndrome) exhibit well-defined female phenotypes and usually go undiscovered until puberty (1/20,000 incidence). The most common cause is a loss of androgen receptors; consequently, these individuals develop female sexual characteristics. However, because they have testes and produce MIS, the paramesonephric duct system is suppressed, and consequently these individuals lack a uterus and oviducts. The testes in these individuals are usually located within the inguinal or labial regions, but there is no spermatogenesis. Unfortunately, about one third of these individuals are likely to develop gonadal malignancies before age 50.

Female pseudohermaphrodites (45, XX) have ovaries and usually have normal internal female reproductive organs; however, they exhibit a malelike external phenotype. This rare anomaly most commonly occurs as a consequence of congenital fetal adrenal hyperplasia, a condition caused by biosynthetic abnormalities that increase the production of androgens and masculinize the external genitalia. The result can range from a slightly enlarged clitoris to development of an almost male-size penis and partially fused labia majora.

21 Appendicular Skeleton and Limb Development

A. Limb Buds and Origins of Cell Types

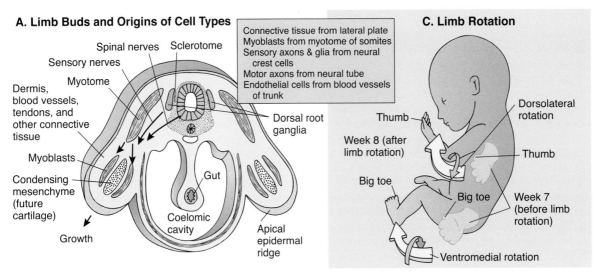

Spinal nerves
Sclerotome
Sensory nerves
Myotome
Dermis, blood vessels, tendons, and other connective tissue
Myoblasts
Condensing mesenchyme (future cartilage)
Growth
Dorsal root ganglia
Gut
Coelomic cavity
Apical epidermal ridge

Connective tissue from lateral plate
Myoblasts from myotome of somites
Sensory axons & glia from neural crest cells
Motor axons from neural tube
Endothelial cells from blood vessels of trunk

C. Limb Rotation

Thumb
Week 8 (after limb rotation)
Big toe
Dorsolateral rotation
Thumb
Week 7 (before limb rotation)
Big toe
Ventromedial rotation

B. Extension of the Limb Buds

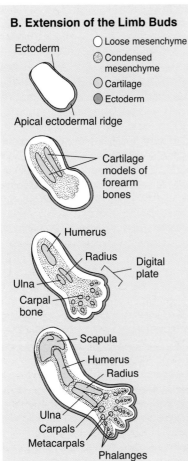

Ectoderm
○ Loose mesenchyme
◎ Condensed mesenchyme
○ Cartilage
● Ectoderm
Apical ectodermal ridge
Cartilage models of forearm bones
Humerus
Radius
Digital plate
Ulna
Carpal bone
Scapula
Humerus
Radius
Ulna
Carpals
Metacarpals
Phalanges

D. Histogenesis of Connective Tissues in the Limbs

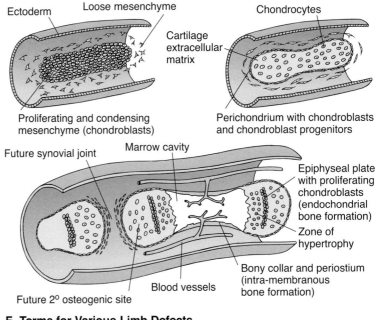

Ectoderm
Loose mesenchyme
Chondrocytes
Cartilage extracellular matrix
Proliferating and condensing mesenchyme (chondroblasts)
Perichondrium with chondroblasts and chondroblast progenitors
Future synovial joint
Marrow cavity
Epiphyseal plate with proliferating chondroblasts (endochondrial bone formation)
Zone of hypertrophy
Bony collar and periostium (intra-membranous bone formation)
Blood vessels
Future 2° osteogenic site

E. Terms for Various Limb Defects

Polydactyly	Extra digits (often dominant inherited trait)
Syndactyly	Fusion of digits (may be fused at bone level; 1/2,200)
Amelia	Absence of 1 or more limbs
Meromelia	Absence of part of a limb
Adactyly	Absence of all digits on a limb
Phocomelia	Short, ill-formed limbs (resemble flippers)
Brachydactyly	Short digits, reduced length of phalanges (often dominant trait; associated with short stature)

OVERVIEW

Limb development begins with formation of an apical epidermal ridge on the limb buds. Somatopleuric mesoderm fills the limb bud and forms the cartilage and bone, connective tissue, tendons and ligaments, and blood vessels of the limb. Skeletal muscles of the limb develop from migrating myotomal cells that invade the limb and are subsequently innervated by corresponding segmental spinal nerves. Most limb anomalies occur as a result of reduction deficits (loss of part of a limb), duplication defects (extra digits), or dysplasias (abnormal tissue amounts). Several genetic and teratogenic mechanisms that cause limb defects have also been identified.

Limb Buds

Limb development begins with proliferation of the lateral plate mesoderm (somatopleuric) in the cervical region (upper limb) and in the lumbar and sacral region (lower limb). This generates small elevations on the ventrolateral body wall. At the tip of each elevation, a thickened ectoderm called the *apical ectodermal ridge* develops (**Part A**). This ridge stimulates the continued proliferation of the underlying mesoderm and is essential for limb formation. As limb buds lengthen, the central mesoderm condenses and differentiates into chondroblasts that form cartilage models of the limb bones (**Parts A** and **B**). The surrounding mesoderm forms the perichondrium, connective tissue, and vasculature of the limb. As the limb bud elongates, the distal end flattens and forms the digital plate, a paddle-shaped structure where digits will form. By day 33 or 34, the hand, forearm, arm, and shoulder regions are distinguishable, and by day 38, mesodermal condensations outlining the fingers can be found within the digital plates. Interdigital cell death (apoptosis) sculpts the fingers from the digital plate. Development of the lower limbs is generally the same except that it is slightly delayed relative to the upper limb.

Initially, both the upper and lower limb buds extend out from the body wall and have their ventral and dorsal surfaces facing the same way as the trunk (**Part C**). However, on about day 51, the upper limbs rotate laterally along their long axis by about 90 degrees. Therefore, the elbows take on a more caudal position, and the original ventral surface of the forearms faces more cranially. By day 54, the lower limbs rotate medially so that the knee faces anteriorly and the original ventral surface faces posteriorly. Therefore, innervation to the limbs becomes twisted along these axes.

Histogenesis of the Connective Tissues in the Limbs

The somatopleuric mesoderm generates the initial core of the limb bud and produces the cartilages, bones, tendons, ligaments, dermis, and vasculature of the limb. As the limb bud elongates, the central mesodermal cells condense and aggregate (**Part B**). These aggregates differentiate into chondrocytes and form cartilage models for all the limb bones (**Parts B** and **D**). Osteogenesis begins in about the seventh week, and bone is deposited around the outer circumference of the cartilage model through intramembranous ossification, forming a bony collar. Meanwhile, some of the central chondrocytes hypertrophy, calcify the surrounding extracellular matrix, and then die. Blood vessels invade this area, bringing in osteoblastic and osteoclastic progenitor cells (**Part D**). The osteoblasts deposit bone on the calcified cartilage to form endochondral bone in areas called *primary ossification centers*. Eventually, endochondral bone is replaced and remodeled into lamellar bone. Endochondral bone formation continues at the ends of long bones in areas called *epiphyseal plates*. Here continued chondroblast proliferation, extracellular matrix deposition, cell hypertrophy, and endochondral bone formation drive the elongation of the bones.

By puberty, however, the entire epiphyseal plate becomes ossified, and bone lengthening ceases. Formation of all the bones of the appendicular skeleton, with exception of a portion of the clavicle, involves endochondral bone formation. Remodeling of the primary ossification sites generates the bone marrow cavities, and these cavities eventually become populated by hematopoietic tissue. Joints form in the mesodermal zones between the chondrogenic rods.

Limb Musculature and Innervation

Skeletal muscles in the limbs are derived from the myotomes at axial levels C5–T1 nd L2–S3. The dermis of the limbs forms from the corresponding dermatomes. Myoblasts migrate into the developing limbs as 2 groups, a dorsal population and a ventral population, and then proliferate and differentiate into skeletal myocytes (**Part A**).

Each somite is associated with a particular spinal nerve, and after exiting the vertebral canal, each nerve divides into dorsal and ventral rami (see Chapters 10 and 31). Limb muscles are innervated by the ventral rami of spinal nerves C5–T1 in the upper limb and L2–S3 in the lower limb. Upon reaching the base of the limb bud, the growth cones combine, sort, and form the brachial and lumbar plexuses seen in the adult through mechanisms not well understood. Upon exiting these plexuses, the nerves go on to establish motor synapses with the developing skeletal muscles. Sensory nerves then follow the motor nerves, using them as guides.

Clinical Aspects

Minor anomalies of the limbs are relatively common and usually can be corrected with surgery. Limb defects are often found as a component of more serious congenital syndromes. Most limb anomalies result from either reduction deficits (loss of part of a limb), duplication defects (extra digits), or dysplasias (abnormal tissue amounts). The terminology used to describe the various types of defects is shown in **Part E**. Many limb defects have a genetic basis. For instance, polydactyly and amelia exhibit autosomal dominant, autosomal recessive, and X-linked patterns of inheritance. Autosomal dominant anomalies include lobster-claw hand and foot, micromelia, and partial tibial defects. Limb defects also are associated with trisomy conditions. Several teratogens target limb development. These include retinoids and anticonvulsants like dimethadione. One of the most powerful teratogens, thalidomide (at one time prescribed as an antinauseant and sedative), causes phocomelia and amelia. Limb defects also can occur in cases of amniotic banding syndrome, whereby strips of torn amniotic membrane wrap around the embryo and fetus and amputate or constrict development of a limb. Limb defects are associated with oligohydramnios (reduced level of amniotic fluid) because this condition prevents the movement of the limbs needed for their normal development. Clubfoot (1/1,000 incidence), a deformity of the foot involving the talus, is one of the most common congenital defects. Affected individuals tend to walk more on their ankles. It is usually corrected surgically.

22 Head and Neck I: Cranial Axial Skeleton and Musculature

A. Skeleton of the Head

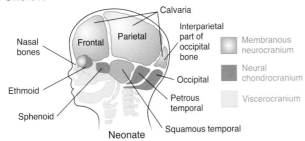

Calvaria
Interparietal part of occipital bone
Frontal
Parietal
Nasal bones
Ethmoid
Sphenoid
Occipital
Petrous temporal
Squamous temporal
Neonate

Membranous neurocranium
Neural chondrocranium
Viscerocranium

B. Viscerocranial Cartilage, Bone, Musculature, and Innervation

Arch	Cartilage	Bones / Ligaments	Origin / Sk. Muscles	Nerve
1	Arch I cartilage (Meckel's)	Intramembranous (maxilla and mandible) Endochondral (incus, malleus) / Sphenomandibular ligament, ligament of malleus	4th somitomere; muscles of mastication, myohyoid, anterior digastric, tensor tympani, tensor veli palatini	CN V
2	Arch II cartilage (Reichert's)	Endochondral (stapes, styloid process, lesser horn and upper rim of hyoid) / Stylohyoid ligaments	6th somitomere; facial muscles, posterior digastric, stylohyoid, stapedius	CN VII
3	Arch III cartilage (hyoid)	Endochondral (greater horn and lower rim of hyoid)	7th somitomere; stylopharyngeus	CN IX
4	Arch IV (laryngeal)		2nd, 3rd, and 4th occipital somites; pharyngeal constrictors, cricothyroid, levator veli palatini	CN X (superior laryngeal)
6	Arch VI (laryngeal)		1st and 2nd occipital somites; intrinsic laryngeal muscles	CN X (recurrent laryngeal)

C. Pharyngeal Arches

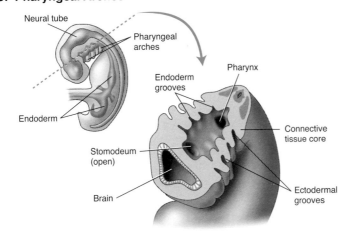

Neural tube
Pharyngeal arches
Endoderm grooves
Pharynx
Endoderm
Connective tissue core
Stomodeum (open)
Brain
Ectodermal grooves

D. Viscerocranial Cartilages and Bones

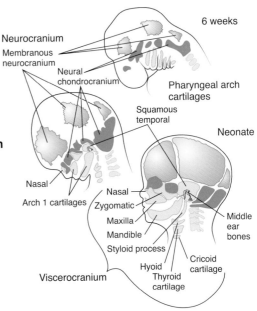

6 weeks
Neurocranium
Membranous neurocranium
Neural chondrocranium
Pharyngeal arch cartilages
Squamous temporal
Neonate
Nasal
Arch 1 cartilages
Nasal
Zygomatic
Maxilla
Mandible
Styloid process
Middle ear bones
Cricoid cartilage
Hyoid
Thyroid cartilage
Viscerocranium

E. Cranial Skeletal Muscle

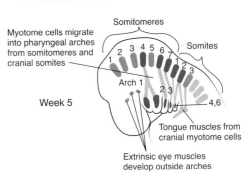

Somitomeres
Myotome cells migrate into pharyngeal arches from somitomeres and cranial somites
Somites
Arch 1
Week 5
Tongue muscles from cranial myotome cells
Extrinsic eye muscles develop outside arches
4,6

F. Cranial Innervation

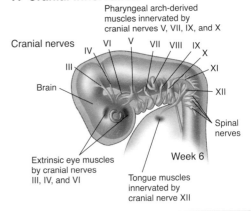

Pharyngeal arch-derived muscles innervated by cranial nerves V, VII, IX, and X
Cranial nerves
IV
V
VI
VII
VIII
IX
X
III
XI
Brain
XII
Spinal nerves
Extrinsic eye muscles by cranial nerves III, IV, and VI
Week 6
Tongue muscles innervated by cranial nerve XII

OVERVIEW

The skull consists of a neurocranium, which covers the brain and sensory organs, and the viscerocranium, which forms the face and surrounds the mouth and upper pharynx. Much of the neurocranium develops via intramembranous bone formation and consists of several different plates that do not completely fuse until late childhood. A large part of the viscerocranium develops from 5 paired pharyngeal arches. Each arch contains an aortic arch vessel, paraxial mesoderm, and neural crest cells, each covered internally by endoderm and externally by ectoderm. Each pharyngeal arch is innervated by a particular cranial nerve. Pharyngeal arch 1 is primarily responsible for development of the maxilla and mandible, a portion of the middle ear, and the associated musculature. Pharyngeal arch 2 forms the stapes, styloid process, and upper part of the hyoid bone and their muscles. Pharyngeal arch 3 forms the greater horn and lower hyoid bone, while pharyngeal arches 4 and 6 contribute to laryngeal structures and laryngeal musculature. Many congenital anomalies of the viscerocranium are related to abnormal morphogenesis of neural crest cells and hypoplasia, including micrognathia, DiGeorge syndrome, and cleft lip and palate.

Skeleton of the Head

The skull is the cranial extension of the axial skeleton. It is divided into 2 parts, the neurocranium, which covers and protects the brain and sense organs, and the viscerocranium, which forms the face and structures surrounding the mouth and leading into the pharynx (**Part A**). The bones of the head are derived from either mesoderm or neural crest cells. The neurocranium is divided into a base called the *chondrocranium* (generated by endochondral ossification) and a calvarial vault called the *membranous neurocranium* (generated by intramembranous ossification) (**Part B**). The bones of the cranial vault are not completely fused at birth but rather have soft fibrous sutures between them that allow continued growth and expansion of the cranial vault during infancy and childhood. Six large fontanelles occupy the corners of the cranial vault at birth. The posterior fontanelles usually close about 3 months after birth, and the superior fontanelle closes by about age 1.5 years. The viscerocranium forms the skeleton of the face and the major parts of the jaw. Most of it develops within pharyngeal arches 1 and 2 (**Part B**).

Pharyngeal Arches

The ventral portion of the head and neck develops bilateral bulges that contain lateral plate mesoderm covered externally by ectoderm and internally by endoderm (**Part C**). Both the outer ectoderm and the inner endoderm form a series of constrictions that almost completely separate the intervening mesenchyme into 5 separate and smaller bulges. These are called the *pharyngeal arches,* each numbered 1 through 4 and 6 (the fifth bulge is a transient structure and never really develops). The intervening endodermally lined outpocketings of the pharynx are called *pharyngeal pouches,* and the external ectodermally lined inpocketings are called *pharyngeal grooves* or *clefts.* Both pharyngeal pouches and grooves develop into important cranial and neck structures that are discussed in Chapter 24. Each pharyngeal arch also contains an aortic arch vessel and is populated by migrating neural crest calls. Therefore, pharyngeal arch mesenchyme is derived from both lateral plate mesoderm and neural crest cells. The neural crest cells form much of the connective tissue found in pharyngeal arches 1, 2, and 3, including their cartilages and bony elements. In contrast, the cartilages in pharyngeal arches 4 and 6 are mesodermally derived.

Viscerocranial Cartilages and Bones

Many of the viscerocranial bones form within pharyngeal arches 1 and 2 (**Part D**). Pharyngeal arch 1 is remodeled into both maxillary and mandibular processes that surround the mouth. In the maxillary process, neural crest cells generate facial and maxillary bones by intramembranous ossification. In the mandibular process, neural crest cells form a cartilage model for the mandibular bone (Meckel's cartilage). Neural crest cells surrounding the cartilage then differentiate into osteoblasts and begin depositing bone on the outside through intramembranous ossification. Much of the cartilage regresses, but a portion undergoes endochondral bone formation to form the incus and malleus (**Part B**). Neural crest cells also form the cartilages found within pharyngeal arches 2 (Reichert's cartilage) and 3 that eventually undergo endochondral bone formation. Reichert's cartilage forms the lesser horn, upper rim of the hyoid bone, and the stapes, while ossification of the cartilages within pharyngeal arch 3 forms the greater horn and lower rim of the hyoid bone. The cartilages within pharyngeal arches 4 and 6 are derived from lateral plate mesoderm rather than neural crest cells. This mesoderm surrounds the endoderm near the developing lung bud and generates the laryngeal cartilages. The surrounding neural crest cells generate the other connective tissue in the area.

Cranial Skeletal Muscle

Each pharyngeal arch develops a functional muscle group derived from somitomeres and occipital somites (**Part E**), and each group is innervated by the cranial nerve associated with that particular pharyngeal arch. As muscle progenitors migrate into the pharyngeal arches, they drag with them the corresponding cranial nerve and continue to do so, although the muscle groups intermingle as they migrate (**Part F**). Therefore, one can identify the adult innervation of the neck and cranial muscles if one recalls the particular pharyngeal arch from which that muscle originated and the cranial nerve associated with that particular pharyngeal arch.

Clinical Aspects

Dysostosis is the term used to describe defective bone development. *Craniofacial dysostosis* refers to anomalies affecting the development of pharyngeal arch 1 and 2 structures and includes mandibulofacial dysostosis (underdevelopment of the lower face), micrognathia (underdeveloped jaw), and components of DiGeorge syndrome (see Chapter 24). Anomalies of the skull range from insignificant minor defects to major defects incompatible with life. Some result from abnormal closure of the skull sutures and others from abnormal growth. One of the more common cranial malformations, craniosynostosis, results from premature closure of the sutures between the major neurocranial bones (1/3,000 live births). Premature closure of the suture between the parietal bones causes scaphocephaly (a long, narrow skull), whereas premature closure of the coronal sutures causes oxycephaly (abnormally high, conical-shaped skull). Some skull defects may be secondary to abnormal brain development, as in the case of anencephaly, microcephaly, and hydrocephaly.

A. Formation of the Face

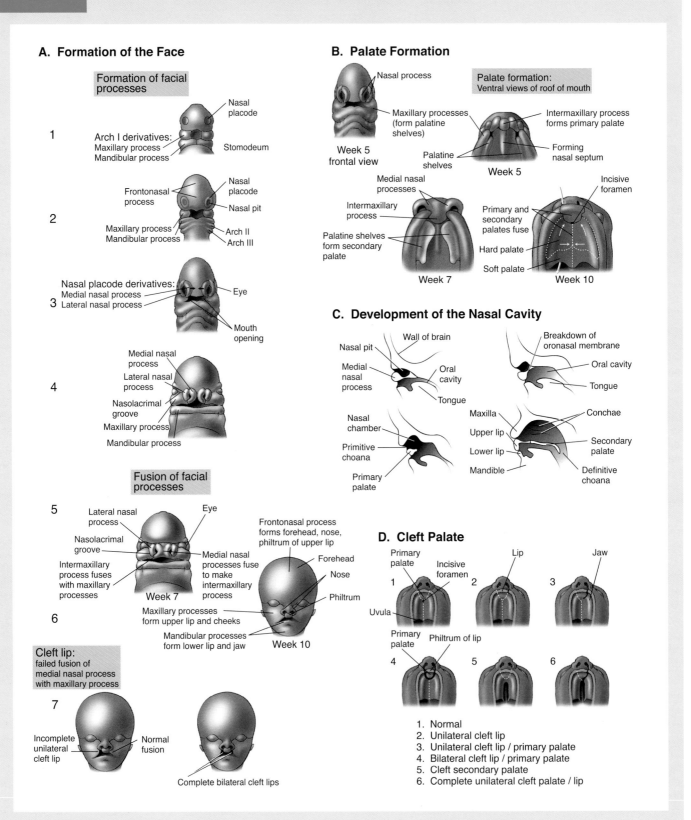

Formation of facial processes

1
Arch I derivatives:
Maxillary process
Mandibular process
Nasal placode
Stomodeum

2
Frontonasal process
Maxillary process
Mandibular process
Nasal placode
Nasal pit
Arch II
Arch III

3
Nasal placode derivatives:
Medial nasal process
Lateral nasal process
Eye
Mouth opening

4
Medial nasal process
Lateral nasal process
Nasolacrimal groove
Maxillary process
Mandibular process

Fusion of facial processes

5
Lateral nasal process
Nasolacrimal groove
Intermaxillary process fuses with maxillary processes
Eye
Medial nasal processes fuse to make intermaxillary process
Week 7

6
Maxillary processes form upper lip and cheeks
Mandibular processes form lower lip and jaw
Frontonasal process forms forehead, nose, philtrum of upper lip
Forehead
Nose
Philtrum
Week 10

Cleft lip:
failed fusion of medial nasal process with maxillary process

7
Incomplete unilateral cleft lip
Normal fusion
Complete bilateral cleft lips

B. Palate Formation

Nasal process
Maxillary processes (form palatine shelves)
Week 5 frontal view

Palate formation:
Ventral views of roof of mouth

Intermaxillary process forms primary palate
Palatine shelves
Forming nasal septum
Week 5

Medial nasal processes
Intermaxillary process
Palatine shelves form secondary palate
Week 7

Incisive foramen
Primary and secondary palates fuse
Hard palate
Soft palate
Week 10

C. Development of the Nasal Cavity

Nasal pit
Wall of brain
Medial nasal process
Oral cavity
Tongue

Breakdown of oronasal membrane
Oral cavity
Tongue

Nasal chamber
Primitive choana
Primary palate

Maxilla
Upper lip
Lower lip
Mandible
Conchae
Secondary palate
Definitive choana

D. Cleft Palate

Primary palate
Incisive foramen
1
Uvula

Lip
2

Jaw
3

Primary palate
Philtrum of lip
4

5

6

1. Normal
2. Unilateral cleft lip
3. Unilateral cleft lip / primary palate
4. Bilateral cleft lip / primary palate
5. Cleft secondary palate
6. Complete unilateral cleft palate / lip

OVERVIEW

The face develops from ectodermally covered mesenchymal processes derived from the first pharyngeal arch and from the frontonasal process surrounding the oral cavity. The enlarging frontonasal process forms a pair of nasal pits surrounded by lateral and medial nasal processes. Fusion of the 2 medial nasal processes generates the intermaxillary process that will form the philtrum and primary palate. The intermaxillary process then fuses with the developing maxillary processes, and together they make the upper lip. Mesenchymal projections extending from the maxillary processes toward the midline fuse with one another to form the secondary palate (the bulk of the adult palate), which in turn fuses with the primary palate. Meanwhile, the paired mandibular processes of pharyngeal arch 1 fuse in the midline to make the mandible. If development of these processes is inadequate or they fail to fuse, facial and palatal defects can result.

Primordia of the Face and Palate

The primordia that form the face appear as bulges developing around the stomodeum (mouth opening) beginning in about the fourth week (**Part A**). These primordia are derivatives of pharyngeal arch 1 and include an unpaired frontonasal process and the paired maxillary and mandibular processes. The bulk of the mesenchyme within these processes is derived from neural crest cells, and growth of these processes is driven by ectodermal-mesenchymal cell interactions resembling those occurring during limb formation. The frontonasal process is associated with forebrain development and consists of a frontal portion (future forehead) and a nasal portion (part between the stomodeum and the forehead). In the fifth week, the paired maxillary processes enlarge and grow ventrally and medially. At the same time, nasal placodes (ectodermal thickenings) form on the inferolateral part of the frontonasal process, invaginate, and form nasal pits. These pits deepen and form the openings of the nasal cavity. Small swellings called *lateral and medial nasal processes* develop on either side of the nasal pit rim. The intervening groove between the lateral nasal process and the maxillary process is called the *nasolacrimal groove*. As these two processes fuse, a solid rod of ectoderm extending the length of the groove remains but eventually canalizes soon after birth, forming the nasolacrimal duct (patency of this duct occurs in about 6% of newborns). The 2 medial nasal processes approach one another and fuse, forming the intermaxillary process. The external portion of the intermaxillary process forms the philtrum and pre-maxillary part of the maxilla. The intermaxillary process then fuses with the maxillary process, and together they make the entire upper lip and maxilla. The intermaxillary process also expands into the oral cavity, forming the primary palate (see below). Meanwhile, the mandibular processes expand and fuse with one another to form the mandible and lower lip. After the first trimester, continued development of the face is primarily limited to changes in the proportions and relative positions of the facial components.

The Palate

Formation of the palate begins at the end of the fifth week, with the most critical period occurring between the sixth and ninth weeks. The intermaxillary process develops a wedge-shaped prominence that projects posteriorly into the oral cavity, forming the primary palate (a small part of the adult hard palate) (**Part B**). Meanwhile 2 mesenchymal projections, the lateral palatine shelves, extend from the maxillary processes toward the midline and fuse with one another to form the secondary palate (bulk of the adult palate). The secondary palate also fuses with the primary palate and developing nasal septum. The bone that develops within the primary palate and anterior part of the secondary palate forms by intramembranous ossification. The posterior portion of the secondary palate forms the soft palate and contains no cartilage or bone. However, it is populated by myoblasts that generate the skeletal muscles important for breathing, swallowing, and vocalization. The incisive foramen marks the fusion point between the primary palate and 2 lateral palatine shelves of the secondary palate.

Nasal Cavity and Olfactory Epithelium

The nasal pits invaginate into the mesenchyme of the frontonasal process and eventually fuse with one another, forming a single nasal cavity that is separated from the developing oral cavity (**Part C**). Eventually, the nasal cavity opens into the developing oral cavity to form an opening called the *primitive choana*. As the secondary palate develops, this opening shifts posteriorly so that the nasal cavity eventually opens into the pharynx. Meanwhile, the frontonasal process develops a midline swelling called the *nasal septum* that extends toward and fuses with the developing primary and secondary palates. Some of the ectodermally derived nasal epithelial cells lining the cavity differentiate into olfactory receptor cells (sensory neurons), whose axons grow into and synapse with secondary neurons in the developing olfactory bulbs.

Clinical Aspects

Complete or partial failure of fusion between any of the swellings results in facial or palatal clefts and may be unilateral or bilateral (**Part D**). Unilateral and bilateral clefts in the palate are usually separated into 3 groups, with the incisive foramen serving as a reference point:

1. Anterior cleft anomalies are clefts anterior to the incisive foramen and include cleft lip with or without fusion between the primary and secondary palates.
2. Posterior clefts are clefts involving the secondary hard and soft palates, resulting from failed fusion of the lateral palatine processes and nasal septum.
3. Complete cleft palates result from a failure of the lateral palatine processes, primary palate, and nasal septum to fuse with one another.

Growth anomalies leading to clefts in the secondary palate usually perturb fusion with the primary palate, thereby leading to anterior clefts as well. If the maxillary processes fail to fuse with lateral and medial nasal processes, an oblique facial cleft extends from the upper lip to the medial margin of the orbit. Cleft lip (1/1,000 births) and cleft palate (1/2,500 births) are common congenital defects. Cleft lips are more common in males than females, but cleft palates are more common in females.

First arch syndrome is a term often used to describe congenital craniofacial anomalies involving the first pharyngeal arch. The etiology is thought to be insufficient development of neural crest cells. Treacher Collins syndrome (mandibulofacial dysostosis) is caused by an autosomal dominant gene leading to a hypoplasia of the zygomatic bones, defects in the lower eyelids, deformed external ears, and sometimes abnormalities of the middle and internal ears. Patients with Pierre Robin syndrome exhibit hypoplasia of the mandible (micrognathia), cleft palate, and defects of the eyes and ears.

24 Head and Neck III: Pharyngeal Arches, Pouches, and Grooves

A. Development of Pharyngeal Pouches and Grooves

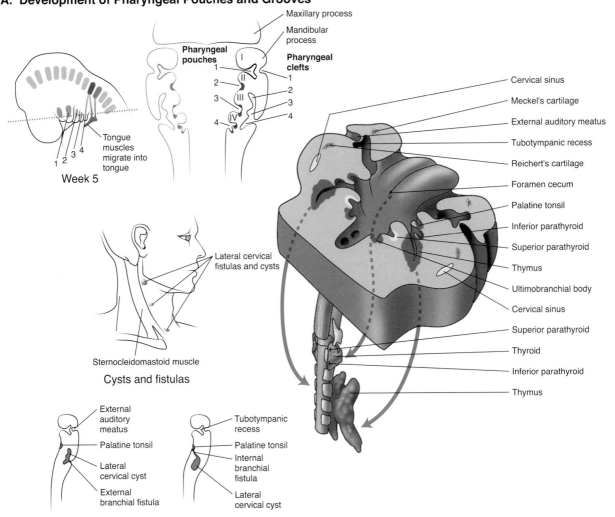

Maxillary process
Mandibular process
Pharyngeal pouches
Pharyngeal clefts
I 1
II 1
2 2
3 III 3
4 IV 4

Tongue muscles migrate into tongue
1 2 3 4

Week 5

Cervical sinus
Meckel's cartilage
External auditory meatus
Tubotympanic recess
Reichert's cartilage
Foramen cecum
Palatine tonsil
Inferior parathyroid
Superior parathyroid
Thymus
Ultimobranchial body
Cervical sinus
Superior parathyroid
Thyroid
Inferior parathyroid
Thymus

Lateral cervical fistulas and cysts

Sternocleidomastoid muscle

Cysts and fistulas

External auditory meatus
Palatine tonsil
Lateral cervical cyst
External branchial fistula

Tubotympanic recess
Palatine tonsil
Internal branchial fistula
Lateral cervical cyst

B. Derivatives of Pharyngeal Pouches and Grooves (clefts)

Pouch / groove	Derivative
Pharyngeal pouch 1 Pharyngeal groove 1	Tubulotympanic recess External auditory meatus
Pharyngeal pouch 2	Palatine tonsil
Pharyngeal pouch 3 　Dorsal 　Ventral	 Inferior parathyroid gland Thymus
Pharyngeal pouch 4 　Dorsal 　Ventral (PP5)	 Superior parathyroid gland Ultimobranchial body (with neural crest → parafollicular C cells)
Pharyngeal grooves 2, 3, and 4	Covered → cervical sinus → obliterated

The ventral portion of the head and neck develops bilateral bulges containing mesoderm and neural crest cells that are covered externally by ectoderm and internally by endoderm. Intervening constrictions form in the mesenchyme, delineating individual pharyngeal arches that are separated from one another by ectodermally lined grooves and endodermally lined pouches. The pharyngeal pouches and grooves generate several important endocrine and immune organs, including the parathyroid glands, thymus, and tonsils. Congenital defects of these tissues and organs can arise as a consequence of abnormal neural crest cell development.

Derivatives of Pharyngeal Pouches and Grooves

The ventral portion of the head and neck develops bilateral bulges containing mesoderm and neural crest cells that are covered externally by ectoderm and internally by endoderm. The pharyngeal arches are delineated within these bulges by invaginations of ectoderm called *pharyngeal grooves* (clefts) and by deep outpocketings of pharyngeal endoderm called *pharyngeal pouches*. The 4 pairs of pharyngeal pouches and grooves are numbered based on the pharyngeal arch found immediately cranial to them (**Part A**). These pouches and grooves form important organs and structures (**Part B**).

Pharyngeal pouch 1 and pharyngeal groove 1 elongate and approach one another, whereas pharyngeal arches 1 and 2 form the maxilla, mandible, and hyoid structures. The endodermally lined pharyngeal pouch 1 forms the middle ear cavity and auditory tube, whereas the ectodermally lined groove forms the epithelium of the external auditory meatus. The remaining intervening tissue becomes the tympanic membrane.

Pharyngeal grooves 2, 3, and 4 do not form adult derivatives. Rather, the second pharyngeal arch overgrows and covers these grooves, forming an ectodermally lined sinus called the *cervical sinus*. This sinus is usually obliterated, but occasionally it remains as a lateral cervical (branchial) cyst. If the second pharyngeal arch fails to completely cover the grooves, a small canal connects the sinus to the exterior surface, forming a cervical (branchial) fistula that usually opens somewhere along the medial-anterior border of the sternocleidomastoid muscle (**Part A**). A cervical fistula usually is discovered because of exterior mucous secretion from the cystic epithelium.

The endodermal lining of pharyngeal pouch 2 proliferates, grows into the mesenchyme, and, together with adjacent mesenchyme, forms the epithelium and stroma of the palatine tonsils. Lymphocytes eventually infiltrate and take up residence in this structure (see Chapter 38).

Pharyngeal pouch 3 expands and splits into dorsal and ventral wings. The dorsal wing forms the inferior parathyroid gland, whereas the ventral wing contributes to the thymus gland. Both glandular primordia lose their connection with the pharynx. The thymic primordium migrates in a caudal and medial direction, pulling the inferior parathyroid primordium with it. As the thymic primordium moves into the thorax, it deposits the inferior parathyroid tissue on the inferior dorsal surface of the developing thyroid gland. The chief (principal) cells of the parathyroid gland that eventually secrete parathyroid hormone and oxyphil cells are derived from the endoderm.

Pharyngeal pouch 4 expands and splits into dorsal and ventral wings. The dorsal wing becomes associated with the caudal or superior surface of the migrating thyroid gland and forms the superior parathyroid gland. The ventral wing divides into 2 smaller outpocketings. The more cranial outpocket is thought to contribute to the thymus gland. The more caudal outpocket, called the *ultimobranchial body,* migrates into the body of the thyroid gland along with neural crest cells. The role of the ultimobranchial body in thyroid gland development is unclear, but parafollicular C-cells (calcitonin-producing cells) found in the adult thyroid are derived from neural crest cells.

Clinical Aspects

DiGeorge syndrome occurs as a consequence of agenesis of the third and fourth pharyngeal pouches. It is characterized by an absence or hypoplasia of the thymus and/or parathyroid glands. Cardiovascular defects and craniofacial anomalies often accompany it. Patients with complete DiGeorge syndrome have immunological deficits, hypocalcemia, and a poor prognosis. Its etiology appears to involve abnormal neural crest development, as these cells play an integral role in the development of all these organs.

25 Head and Neck IV: Tongue, Thyroid, and Pituitary Gland

A. Tongue Development

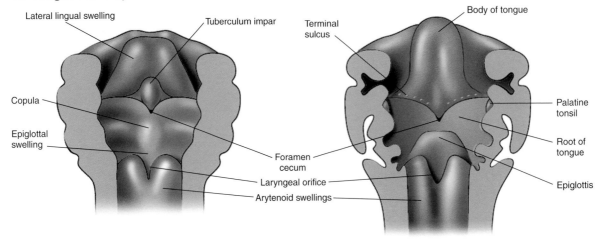

Lateral lingual swelling
Tuberculum impar
Copula
Epiglottal swelling
Foramen cecum
Laryngeal orifice
Arytenoid swellings

Terminal sulcus
Body of tongue
Palatine tonsil
Root of tongue
Epiglottis

B. Thyroid Gland Development

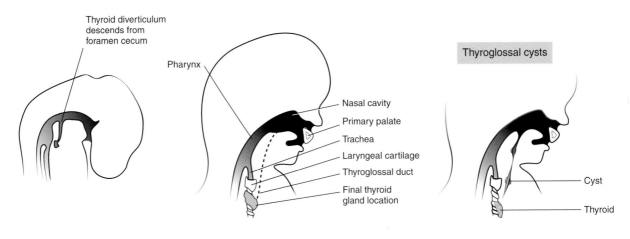

Thyroid diverticulum descends from foramen cecum

Pharynx

Nasal cavity
Primary palate
Trachea
Laryngeal cartilage
Thyroglossal duct
Final thyroid gland location

Thyroglossal cysts

Cyst
Thyroid

C. Pituitary Gland Development

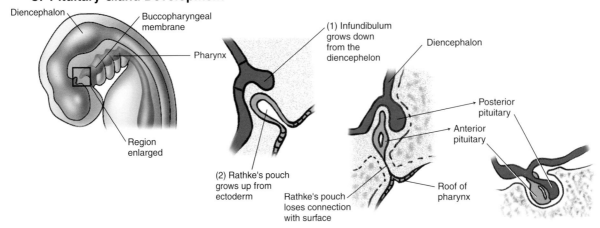

Diencephalon
Buccopharyngeal membrane
Pharynx
Region enlarged

(1) Infundibulum grows down from the diencephelon
(2) Rathke's pouch grows up from ectoderm
Rathke's pouch loses connection with surface

Diencephalon
Posterior pituitary
Anterior pituitary
Roof of pharynx

OVERVIEW

The bilateral sets of pharyngeal arches fuse in the ventral midline, forming a primitive oral and pharyngeal cavity. The fusion of the endodermally covered mesenchymal swellings on the floor of the oral cavity generates the tongue, while an endodermal diverticulum between pharyngeal arches 1 and 2 generates the thyroid gland. The pituitary gland develops from a diencephalic diverticulum and Rathke's pouch, an ectodermal diverticulum forming just outside the oral cavity. Remnants of the thyroglossal diverticulum and duct and aberrant remnants of Rathke's pouch can lead to the formation of cysts, fistulas, and tumors.

Tongue Development

The tongue develops through the formation, growth, and fusion of mesenchymal swellings projecting into the oral cavity from the first 4 pharyngeal arches (**Part A**). It is covered by epithelium derived from pharyngeal endoderm, contains connective tissue derived from neural crest cells, and is composed of muscle derived from the first 3 occipital somites (innervated by cranial nerve XII). Some of the overlying endodermal cells differentiate into taste buds (innervated by special sensory nerves from cranial nerve VII). Tongue development begins in the fourth week when the first pharyngeal arch forms a median swelling called the *tuberculum impar*. Concurrently, lateral lingual swellings form on both sides and eventually overgrow the median swelling. Collectively, these 3 swellings form the anterior two thirds of the tongue, and because they are derived from pharyngeal arch 1, the sensory innervation is carried by cranial nerve V. Meanwhile, median swellings form in pharyngeal arch 2 (the copula) and in pharyngeal arches 3 and 4 (the hypobranchial eminence). The hypobranchial eminence overgrows the copula and forms the posterior one third of tongue. Because pharyngeal arch 3 is the largest contributor to this portion of the tongue, it is mostly innervated by cranial nerve IX (the cranial nerve of pharyngeal arch 3) with some innervation from cranial nerve X. The boundary between the anterior and posterior tongue is demarcated by a depression called the *foramen cecum*, the site of thyroid gland development.

Thyroid Gland Development

Late in the fourth week, the endoderm of the foramen cecum proliferates and forms the thyroid primordium (**Part B**). This primordium descends in front of the foregut and remains connected to the tongue by a narrow canal called the *thyroglossal duct* that eventually disappears. The developing thyroid gland descends in front of the hyoid bone and laryngeal cartilages and reaches its final position in front of the trachea during week 7. By this time, it has acquired an isthmus and 2 lobes. At the end of the first trimester, thyroid follicular cells (derived from the endoderm) begin producing colloid, the stored form of thyroxine and triiodothyronine. The connective tissue of the thyroid gland and the parafollicular C-cells are derived from neural crest cells.

Pituitary Gland Development

The pituitary gland develops from 2 different structures, the Rathke pouch and the infundibulum of the diencephalon (**Part C**). The Rathke pouch is an ectodermal inpocketing that appears in front of the buccopharyngeal membrane during the third week. This pouch grows dorsally toward the infundibulum of the diencephalon and by the end of the eighth week loses its connection with the exterior. The Rathke pouch forms the anterior pituitary gland. The infundibulum develops as a downward diverticulum from the third ventricle of the diencephalon and forms the pituitary stalk and posterior pituitary gland (see also Chapter 30).

Clinical Aspects

Thyroglossal cysts can form if the thyroglossal duct does not regress (**Part B**). If these cysts are connected to the outside, they form a thyroglossal fistula. Thyroglossal cysts can be found anywhere along the path of thyroid migration, but 50% of the time they are located close to or just inferior to the hyoid bone. Aberrant thyroid tissue also may be found along this path and is subject to the same diseases as the gland itself. Similarly, remnants of the Rathke pouch can persist in the roof of the pharynx, forming accessory pituitary tissue called a *pharyngeal hypophysis*. These remnants can sometimes develop into tumors called *craniopharyngiomas*.

26 The Eye

A. Progenitors of the Eye

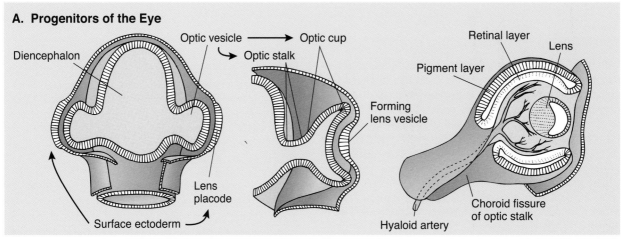

Diencephalon

Optic vesicle → Optic cup

↘ Optic stalk

Lens placode

Surface ectoderm

Forming lens vesicle

Retinal layer

Lens

Pigment layer

Hyaloid artery

Choroid fissure of optic stalk

B. Optic Cup and Surrounding Tissues

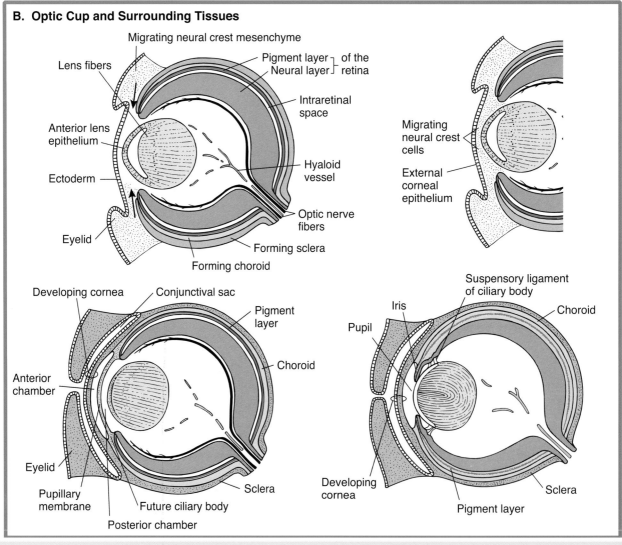

Migrating neural crest mesenchyme

Lens fibers

Pigment layer ⎤ of the
Neural layer ⎦ retina

Intraretinal space

Anterior lens epithelium

Hyaloid vessel

Ectoderm

Optic nerve fibers

Eyelid

Forming sclera

Forming choroid

Migrating neural crest cells

External corneal epithelium

Developing cornea

Conjunctival sac

Pigment layer

Choroid

Anterior chamber

Eyelid

Pupillary membrane

Future ciliary body

Posterior chamber

Sclera

Suspensory ligament of ciliary body

Iris

Choroid

Pupil

Developing cornea

Sclera

Pigment layer

OVERVIEW

Eye development begins with the formation of bilateral extensions from the forebrain. These grow toward the ectoderm and form optic vesicles on the distal end of long optic stalks. Each optic vesicle invaginates, forming the bilayered optic cup. The outer layer of the optic cup forms the outer pigmented layer of the retina, and the inner layer forms the neural retina and membranes of the iris and choroid body. The optic vesicle induces formation of a lens vesicle from the ectoderm. The lens vesicle eventually forms the lens and lies posterior to the developing iris. The surrounding mesoderm-derived and neural crest-derived mesenchyme forms the choroid, sclera, corneal fibroblasts, and skeletal muscles.

Early Development

Development of each eye begins with the formation of lateral out-pocketings from both sides of the early diencephalon called the *optic vesicles* (**Part A**). As the optic vesicles approach the surface ectoderm, they invaginate so that one side of the vesicle touches the other side. This forms a 2-layered optic cup that remains attached to the diencephalon by the optic stalk (future optic nerve). While the 2 layers appose one another and attach, the attachment is never firm and they can be easily separated. The invagination forming the optic cup also extends along the optic stalk, forming the choroid fissure. The developing hyaloid artery and vein (which will form the central artery and vein of the retina) become incorporated into this fissure and eventually are fully enveloped by the optic stalk. Meanwhile, the optic vesicle or cup induces overlying ectoderm to form a lens placode. This placode invaginates to form the optic pit, which later separates from the ectoderm, forming the lens vesicle and, later, the lens.

The Optic Cup

The outer layer of the optic cup forms retinal pigmented epithelium, whereas the inner layer differentiates into the multilayered neural retina, iris, and ciliary body (**Part B**). The posterior four fifths of the inner layer differentiates into multiple layers, the photoreceptive layer (rods and cones) and a mantle layer (outer and inner nuclear layers and ganglion layer). The anterior-most one fifth contributes to the iris and ciliary body. Because the retinal portion of the optic vesicle invaginates, epithelial cells of the neural retina are inverted (i.e., light must first pass through the entire base of the retinal layer before reaching the apical photoreceptive ends of the rods and cones). Myelination of the optic nerve fibers is incomplete at the time of birth but is completed usually within 10 weeks after the eyes have been exposed to light. During development of the optic cup, a loose mesenchyme fills the cavity of the cup, and these cells secrete a gelatinous material called the *vitreous body*. The distal hyaloid artery supplies this area and the early lens. Later in development, the distal segments of the hyaloid vessels regress, but the proximal portions remain as the central vessels of the optic stalk. However, if parts of the distal hyaloid vessels persist, they can form cords or cysts in the area of the optic disk.

Outer Layers

During weeks 6 and 7, the mesenchyme surrounding the optic cup differentiates into 2 layers, an inner pigmented vascular layer called the *choroid* and an outer fibrous layer called the *sclera* (**Part B**). Cornea formation is induced by the lens. Ectoderm overlying the newly formed lens differentiates into the external corneal epithelium and begins depositing extracellular matrix between it and the lens. During the seventh week, neural crest cells migrate along this extracellular matrix, filling it with mesenchyme. This mesenchyme splits into 2 layers, forming an intervening cavity (the anterior chamber). Neural crest cells lining the anterior surface of the anterior chamber differentiate into corneal endothelial cells, and those between the corneal endothelium and external corneal epithelium form corneal fibroblasts.

The posterior chamber develops by a cavitation of the neural crest-derived mesenchyme remaining in front of the lens. Neural crest mesenchymal cells between the posterior chamber and anterior chamber form a temporary membrane called the *pupillary membrane*. Meanwhile, the anterior rim of the optic cup, consisting of the fused pigmented and retinal layers, expands and slightly overlaps the lens. The pupil forms when the papillary membrane ruptures, thereby connecting the anterior and posterior chambers. The remaining pupillary cells, now adjacent to the anterior rim, differentiate into the connective tissue of the iris, the dilator and sphincter pupillary muscles, and the ciliary process. Ciliary muscles focusing the lens are also derived from neural crest cells.

Extrinsic Structures

The extrinsic muscles of the eye are derived from the first 3 somitomeres and are innervated by cranial nerves III, IV, and VI. The eyelids form from 2 folds of ectoderm filled with neural crest mesenchyme that extend from above and below the cornea. The upper and lower eyelids fuse to one another beginning in the 10th week and remain so until the 26th week. During this time, the space between the lids and cornea expands to form the conjunctival sac, and, when the lids reopen, a part of the ectoderm now overlies the sclera (bulbar conjunctiva). The ectoderm lining the inner eyelid is called the *palpebral conjunctiva*. The myoblasts that migrate into the eyelids are derived from pharyngeal arch 2 and therefore are innervated by cranial nerve VII. The lacrimal glands develop from the ectodermal buds invaginating into the eyelid that subsequently differentiate into alveolar gland cells and ducts.

Clinical Aspects

During development of the eye, failure of the choroid fissure to close produces a dark notch (cleft) within the iris called *coloboma of the iris*. This condition is relatively common and is sometimes transmitted as an autosomal dominant trait. If the inner and outer layers of the optic cup do not attach to each other, a congenital detached retina results. Usually the lens is transparent, but occasionally it remains opaque, causing congenital cataracts. This condition can be inherited or caused by maternal rubella virus infection or exposure to radiation. Congenital glaucoma, an abnormal development of the drainage system for aqueous humor, may also occur as a consequence of a rubella infection or may be inherited via recessive mutant genes.

Microphthalmos, having a very small or underdeveloped eye, usually accompanies other craniofacial anomalies or appears as part of a syndrome. Cytomegalovirus infection or toxoplasmosis also can increase the risk of developing this anomaly. Cryptophthalmos is the congenital absence of the eyelids and may be inherited as an autosomal recessive trait. Anophthalmos is a congenital absence of the entire eye, but eyelids may still form.

27 The Ear

A. Primordia of the Inner Ear

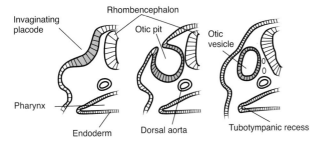

- Invaginating placode
- Rhombencephalon
- Otic pit
- Otic vesicle
- Pharynx
- Endoderm
- Dorsal aorta
- Tubotympanic recess

B. Development of Inner and Middle Ear

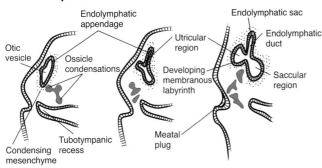

- Endolymphatic appendage
- Endolymphatic sac
- Otic vesicle
- Ossicle condensations
- Utricular region
- Endolymphatic duct
- Developing membranous labyrinth
- Saccular region
- Condensing mesenchyme
- Tubotympanic recess
- Meatal plug

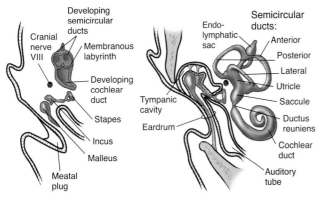

- Developing semicircular ducts
- Cranial nerve VIII
- Membranous labyrinth
- Developing cochlear duct
- Stapes
- Incus
- Malleus
- Meatal plug
- Endolymphatic sac
- Semicircular ducts:
  - Anterior
  - Posterior
  - Lateral
- Utricle
- Saccule
- Ductus reuniens
- Cochlear duct
- Tympanic cavity
- Eardrum
- Auditory tube

C. Development of the Cochlear Duct

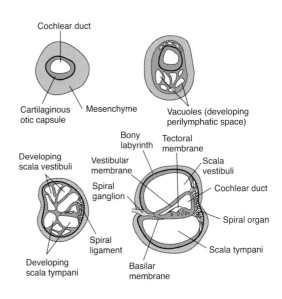

- Cochlear duct
- Cartilaginous otic capsule
- Mesenchyme
- Vacuoles (developing perilymphatic space)
- Developing scala vestibuli
- Bony labyrinth
- Tectoral membrane
- Vestibular membrane
- Scala vestibuli
- Spiral ganglion
- Cochlear duct
- Spiral organ
- Spiral ligament
- Scala tympani
- Developing scala tympani
- Basilar membrane

D. Development of the Vestibular System

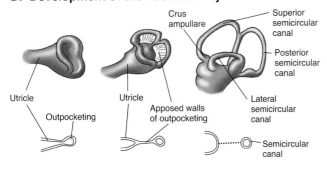

- Crus ampullare
- Superior semicircular canal
- Posterior semicircular canal
- Lateral semicircular canal
- Utricle
- Outpocketing
- Apposed walls of outpocketing
- Semicircular canal

E. Development of the External Ear

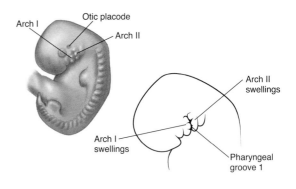

- Otic placode
- Arch I
- Arch II
- Arch II swellings
- Arch I swellings
- Pharyngeal groove 1

6 auricular swellings form around pharyngeal groove 1:

Arch 1 (1-3)   Arch 2 (4-6)

Auricular swellings fuse:

OVERVIEW

Development of the ear begins with the formation and invagination of bilateral ectodermal pits on either side of the rhombencephalon. These otic pits separate from the ectoderm and form the otic vesicles that are remodeled into the membranous labyrinth of the inner ear. Each otic vesicle forms a saccule, utricle, semicircular canals, and cochlear duct. Mesenchyme surrounding the membranous labyrinth differentiates into cartilage, and in the area of the cochlear duct, this cartilage vacuolizes to generate the scala vestibuli and scala tympani. The middle ear cavity and auditory tube form from an expansion of the first pharyngeal pouch and are lined with endoderm. The middle ear cavity portion expands and envelops the developing middle ear bones. The external acoustic meatus develops from a medial extension of the first pharyngeal groove. Ectoderm-covered swellings of mesenchyme surrounding the external acoustic meatus generate auricular hillocks that eventually become the auricle of the ear. Congenital deafness may occur as a result of abnormal development of the membranous and bony labyrinths or because of defects in the development of the auditory ossicles or eardrum. Defects of the external ear are also common.

Inner Ear

Ear development begins with the formation of ectodermal placodes called the *otic placodes* that develop lateral to the rhombencephalic neural tube on about day 22 (**Part A**). These placodes quickly form pits that eventually separate from the surface, generating the otic (auditory) vesicles. Each otic vesicle is remodeled into a ventral component (forms the saccule and cochlear duct) and dorsal component (forms the utricle, semicircular canals, and endolymphatic duct) collectively known as the *membranous labyrinth* (**Part B**). This membranous labyrinth accumulates a fluid called *endolymph*. Beginning in the fifth week, a long spiraling extension of the saccule develops, and this epithelium differentiates into the cochlear duct. Meanwhile, the mesenchyme surrounding the cochlear duct begins differentiating into cartilage, forming an otic capsule that later ossifies (**Part C**). During the early fetal period, cartilage adjacent to the cochlear duct vacuolizes, creating 2 cavities that become filled with fluid (perilymph) and surround the cochlear duct. These are the scala vestibuli and scala tympani. The remaining mesenchyme adjacent to the cochlear duct contributes to the vestibular and basilar membranes and anchors the cochlear duct medially (spiral lamina) and laterally (spiral ligament) to the future bony labyrinth. Meanwhile, the epithelium of the cochlear duct adjacent to the basilar membrane develops 2 ridges. Cells in the lateral ridge differentiate into the outer hair cells, whereas cells in the medial ridge differentiate into the inner hair cells. The cilia of these hair cells become embedded in a gelatinous membrane called the *tectorial membrane* that forms within the cochlear duct and is attached to its inner wall. Together with the hair cells, the tectorial membrane makes up the organ of Corti. Hair cells are the sensory cells that transduce mechanical vibrations, initially produced by sound, into electrical signals. These signals are transmitted to sensory ganglion cells found along the cochlear duct (spiral ganglion) and belonging to the eighth cranial nerve.

The semicircular canals form from flattened outpocketings of the utricular portion of the otic vesicles (**Part D**). As they flatten, the sides of the outpockets become apposed to one another other and fuse, and the central segment disappears. What remains is a series of hollow outer loops that differentiate into the semicircular canals. At the base of each canal where they meet the utricle, the semicircular canals dilate and develop specialized sensory structures called the *crista ampullari* that protrude into the membranous labyrinth. These structures transduce changes in angular acceleration into electrical signals. Similar structures develop within the utricle and saccule and serve as detectors of body orientation. The vestibular portion of cranial nerve VIII innervates these sensory organs. During early development of the utricle, the utricle forms a long extending diverticulum called the *endolymphatic duct*. This duct is involved in removing excess endolymphatic fluid from the inner membranous labyrinth.

Middle Ear

As discussed in Chapter 24, the tympanic cavity forms from the first pharyngeal pouch and is lined with endoderm. This extension of the first pharyngeal pouch is called the *tubotympanic recess*. This recess widens at the distal end to form the middle ear cavity (tympanic cavity) and narrows at the proximal end to form the auditory (eustachian) tube (**Part B**). The malleus and incus ossicles are derived from cartilage models originating in the first pharyngeal arch, while the stapes forms within the second pharyngeal arch. These bones remain embedded within the mesenchyme, but during the eighth month the tympanic cavity expands and envelops these bones. The muscle of malleus forms from the first pharyngeal arch mesoderm and therefore is innervated by cranial nerve V (cranial nerve of the first pharyngeal arch). The stapedius muscle is derived from second pharyngeal arch mesoderm and is innervated by cranial nerve VII (cranial nerve of the second pharyngeal arch).

External Ear

The external auditory meatus is generated from the first pharyngeal groove. Ectoderm from this groove grows medially as a solid cord (meatal plug) that later recanalizes (**Part B**). The tympanic membrane (eardrum) forms from apposition of the endodermally lined tympanic cavity (first pharyngeal pouch) and the ectodermally lined external auditory meatus plus a small amount of intervening connective tissue. The auricle of the ear develops from 6 mesenchymal projections, called *auricular hillocks,* surrounding the exterior of the first pharyngeal groove (**Part E**). The auricular hillocks expand, fuse, and make the final auricle. Neural crest cells provide much of the mesenchyme comprising these hillocks.

Clinical Aspects

Congenital deafness can occur as result of abnormal development of the membranous and bony labyrinths. Maternal rubella infection during the seventh and eighth weeks of pregnancy can damage the developing organ of Corti. Congenital deafness also can occur as a consequence of abnormal development of the auditory ossicles or eardrum. Such malformations often accompany craniofacial defects, including first arch syndrome. Sometimes the meatal plug does not canalize, leading to atresia of the external acoustic meatus, and, in most cases, meatal atresia is associated with first arch syndrome. Defects in the development of the external ear often accompany other congenital anomalies and serve as indicators that the infant should be examined more closely for other defects. *Anotia* is the absence of an auricle. *Microtia* is the term for a small or rudimentary auricle.

28 Nervous System I: Early Development and the Spinal Cord

A. Early Neural Tube

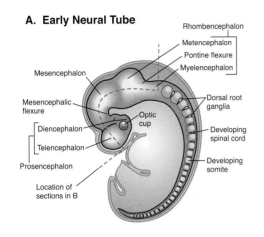

- Rhombencephalon
- Metencephalon
- Pontine flexure
- Myelencephalon
- Mesencephalon
- Mesencephalic flexure
- Optic cup
- Diencephalon
- Telencephalon
- Prosencephalon
- Location of sections in B
- Dorsal root ganglia
- Developing spinal cord
- Developing somite

B. Brain Ventricles

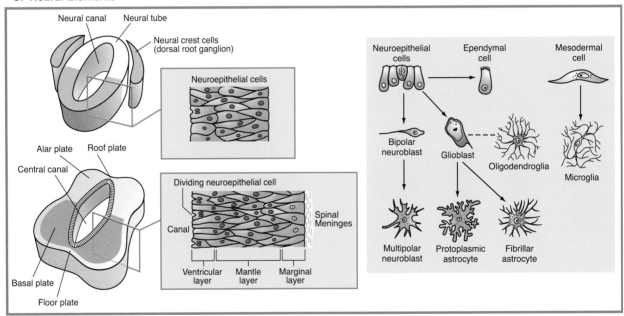

3 primary vesicles
- Wall
- Cavity
- Forebrain (prosencephalon)
- Midbrain (mesencephalon)
- Hindbrain (rhombencephalon)

5 secondary vesicles
- Telencephalon
- Diencephalon
- Mesencephalon
- Metencephalon
- Myelencephalon
- Spinal cord

Adult derivatives of

walls	cavities
Cerebral hemispheres	Lateral ventricles
Thalami, etc.	3rd ventricle*
Midbrain	Cerebral aqueduct of Sylvius
Pons	Upper part of 4th ventricle
Cerebellum	
Medulla	Lower part of 4th ventricle

* Cranial 1/3 from telencephalon

C. Neural Elements

- Neural canal
- Neural tube
- Neural crest cells (dorsal root ganglion)
- Neuroepithelial cells
- Alar plate
- Roof plate
- Central canal
- Dividing neuroepithelial cell
- Canal
- Spinal Meninges
- Basal plate
- Floor plate
- Ventricular layer
- Mantle layer
- Marginal layer

- Neuroepithelial cells
- Ependymal cell
- Mesodermal cell
- Bipolar neuroblast
- Glioblast
- Oligodendroglia
- Microglia
- Multipolar neuroblast
- Protoplasmic astrocyte
- Fibrillar astrocyte

D. Spinal Cord Organization

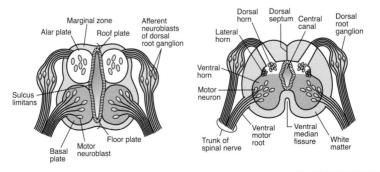

- Alar plate
- Marginal zone
- Roof plate
- Afferent neuroblasts of dorsal root ganglion
- Sulcus limitans
- Basal plate
- Motor neuroblast
- Floor plate

- Dorsal horn
- Dorsal septum
- Central canal
- Dorsal root ganglion
- Lateral horn
- Ventral horn
- Motor neuron
- Trunk of spinal nerve
- Ventral motor root
- Ventral median fissure
- White matter

OVERVIEW

The neural tube becomes delineated into 5 regions along the cranial-caudal axis: the telencephalon and diencephalon, the mesencephalon, the metencephalon, the myelencephalon, and the spinal cord. Proliferating neuroepithelial cells form neuroblasts (future neurons), then glioblasts (future astrocytes and oligodendrocytes), and then ependymal cells. Neuroblasts become organized into ventricular (mitotic layer), mantle (neuroblasts and glia), and marginal (nerve fibers and glia) layers. Neuroblasts aggregate and form a ventral and dorsal column of cells running along the length of the spinal cord. Cells in the ventral column differentiate into somatic motor neurons, and their axons exit via the ventral spinal root. Cells in the dorsal column differentiate into association neurons that receive sensory input from the periphery via the dorsal root ganglia.

Early Neural Tube

Development of the nervous system begins with the formation of the ectodermally derived neural tube. This tube initially develops 3 different expansions at the cranial end: the prosencephalon (forebrain), mesencephalon (midbrain), and rhombencephalon (hindbrain) (**Part A**). Meanwhile, 2 flexures develop within the neural tube as a consequence of embryonic growth, one in the midbrain region (the midbrain flexure) and the other between the hindbrain and future spinal cord (the cervical flexure). The forebrain develops 2 lateral outpocketings (the telencephalon) projecting from a central vesicle (the diencephalon). The telencephalon will form the cerebral hemispheres. The diencephalon will form the thalamus, hypothalamus, posterior pituitary, and optic vesicles. Meanwhile, the hindbrain organizes into 2 regions, the metencephalon (which forms the pons and cerebellum) and the myelencephalon (which forms the medulla oblongata).

Brain Ventricles

With the dilatation and expansion of the neural tube, the luminal compartments within each cranial segment develop into cavities called *ventricles* (**Part B**). These ventricles are continuous with one another and with the central canal of the developing spinal cord. The cavities within the expanding telencephalon form the lateral ventricles of the brain, while the cavity within the diencephalon forms most of the third ventricle. Communication between the lateral ventricles and the third ventricle is through an opening called the *foramen of Monro*. The cavity within the hindbrain forms the fourth ventricle and is connected to the third ventricle by means of a small midbrain cavity (the cerebral aqueduct of Sylvius). A specialized complex called the *choroid plexus* forms within the ependymal layer lining the ventricles (discussed below).

Development of the Neural Elements

The initial organization and cellular differentiation of the neural tube in the spinal cord and brain are similar. Once formed, the wall of the neural tube consists of pseudostratified neuroepithelial cells that are connected to one another by specialized junctions at the luminal ends. As the neural tube closes, the neuroepithelial cells begin dividing, forming neuroblasts (future neurons). As the neuroepithelial cells enter mitosis, they retract toward the luminal side of the neural tube, generating a layer of mitotic cells called the *ventricular layer* (**Part C**). As the number of neuroblasts increase, they begin aggregating and residing in a separate layer just outside the ventricular layer. This is called the *mantle layer*. The neuroblasts within the mantle layer begin differentiating into neurons, and these neurons extend nerve fibers. As these nerve fibers extend up and down the neural axis, they form another layer outside the mantle layer, called the *marginal layer*. Nerve fibers in the marginal layer eventually become myelinated to form the white matter of the spinal cord.

The neuroepithelial cells then begin producing a new cell type called *glioblasts*. Glioblasts differentiate into astrocytes and oligodendrocytes.

Finally, neuroepithelial cells produce the ependymal cells that line the lumen of the spinal cord and brain, and these cells are responsible for producing CSF. Later in development, a third type of glial cell called *microglia* appears. Microglia are phagocytic cells that serve as the scavenger cells for the central nervous system. Microglia are derived from mesoderm cells entering the central nervous system during its vascularization.

Spinal Cord Organization

As the neuroblasts within the mantle layer increase in number, they organize into ventral and dorsal columns on either side of the developing spinal cord (**Part D**). The ventral aggregates, called *basal plates*, differentiate into somatic motor neurons of the ventral horn. These neurons eventually develop axons that exit the spinal cord, forming the ventral roots of the spinal nerves, and innervate voluntary muscles (general somatic efferents). The dorsal aggregates form the alar plates. These neuroblasts differentiate into association neurons (interneurons) that interconnect the motor neurons of the basal plate with the sensory neurons of the developing dorsal root ganglia. As plate development progresses, the dorsal and ventral neuroepithelium thins in the midline, forming the roof and floor plates that eventually serve as commissures for nerve fibers. Neuroblasts also aggregate between the ventral and dorsal horns at spinal levels T1–L2/L3 and S2–S4, forming the intermediate or lateral horn. These cells differentiate into the sympathetic and sacral parasympathetic preganglionic neurons (general visceral efferent) (see Chapter 31). These neurons project their axons out of the spinal cord via the ventral roots.

The Meninges

The mesenchyme immediately surrounding the neural tube condenses to form membranous-like tissues called the *primordial meninx*. The outer portion of this membrane differentiates into the dura mater, while the inner portion forms the leptomeninges. The leptomeninges is further subdivided into the arachnoid mater and pia mater by the formation of a fluid-filled space called the *subarachnoid space*. Mesenchymal cells forming the dura mater and the leptomeninges are derived from mesoderm, with the exception that the part of the forebrain and midbrain leptomeninges is of neural crest origin.

Clinical Aspects

Hydrocephaly is a condition whereby abnormal levels of CSF accumulate within the brain, leading to enlargement of the ventricles, brain, and skull. It can be caused by an imbalance between the production and removal of CSF or by a blockage or stenosis of the communications between the brain ventricles. Arnold-Chiari malformation is hydrocephalus caused by an overgrown cerebellum protruding and blocking the flow of CSF through the foramen magnum. Some of the other neural tube and spinal cord defects are described in Chapter 9.

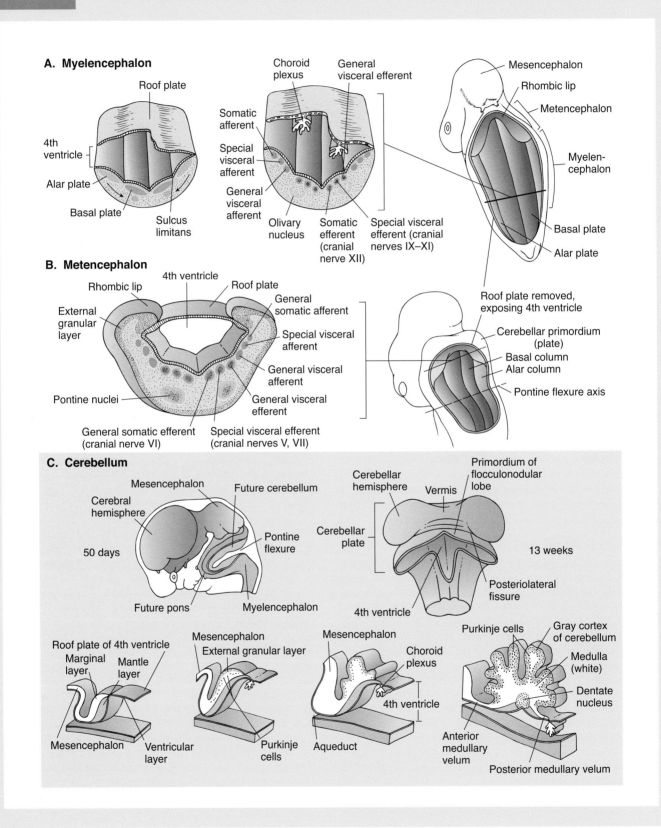

A. Myelencephalon

Roof plate

4th ventricle

Alar plate

Basal plate

Sulcus limitans

Choroid plexus

General visceral efferent

Somatic afferent

Special visceral afferent

General visceral afferent

Olivary nucleus

Somatic efferent (cranial nerve XII)

Special visceral efferent (cranial nerves IX–XI)

Mesencephalon

Rhombic lip

Metencephalon

Myelen-cephalon

Basal plate

Alar plate

B. Metencephalon

Rhombic lip

4th ventricle

Roof plate

External granular layer

General somatic afferent

Special visceral afferent

General visceral afferent

General visceral efferent

Pontine nuclei

General somatic efferent (cranial nerve VI)

Special visceral efferent (cranial nerves V, VII)

Roof plate removed, exposing 4th ventricle

Cerebellar primordium (plate)

Basal column

Alar column

Pontine flexure axis

C. Cerebellum

Mesencephalon

Cerebral hemisphere

Future cerebellum

Pontine flexure

50 days

Future pons

Myelencephalon

Cerebellar hemisphere

Vermis

Primordium of flocculonodular lobe

Cerebellar plate

Posteriolateral fissure

4th ventricle

13 weeks

Roof plate of 4th ventricle

Marginal layer

Mantle layer

Mesencephalon

Ventricular layer

Mesencephalon

External granular layer

Purkinje cells

Mesencephalon

Choroid plexus

4th ventricle

Aqueduct

Purkinje cells

Gray cortex of cerebellum

Medulla (white)

Dentate nucleus

Anterior medullary velum

Posterior medullary velum

OVERVIEW

The organization of the hindbrain (i.e., alar plate and basal plate) is very similar to that in the spinal cord. However, in the hindbrain the roof plate widens and thins so that the alar plate becomes more lateral relative to the basal plate. As in the spinal cord, the alar plates of the myelencephalon and metencephalon are primarily associated with generating sensory nuclei, whereas the basal plates primarily generate the motor nuclei. But in the hindbrain, these nuclei contribute extensively to the sensory and motor components of cranial nerves V–XII. The myelencephalon also forms the medulla oblongata. The metencephalon forms the pons and cerebellum, important for controlling posture, movement, balance, and hearing. Additional cell layers within the cerebellum form by proliferation of neuroblasts within the mantle layer, followed by subsequent migration into the cortex, more proliferation, and subsequent differentiation.

Organization of the Brain Segment of the Neural Tube

The neuroepithelium of the spinal cord organizes into 3 basic layers, the ventricular layer, mantle layer, and marginal layer. These 3 layers are retained in the brainstem portion of the neural tube, but in the more cranial regions of the brain, they expand into 5 layers through a proliferation and migration of neuroblasts. Like the spinal cord, the alar and basal plates develop within the brain, but the shape of the neural tube is remodeled such that the alar plates become more lateral than dorsal to the basal plate (**Part A**). In addition, the roof of the neural tube becomes thinner and wider, particularly in the areas of the myelencephalon, metencephalon, and mesencephalon. In the developing prosencephalon, the alar plates become greatly accentuated, and the basal plate practically disappears. During this process, differentiating neuroblasts migrate, aggregate, and organize into groups referred to as *nuclei* within the developing brain. As in the spinal cord, the alar groups generate neurons primarily associated with receiving and transmitting sensory information, whereas the basal groups are primarily associated with motor functions. Some of the alar and basal groups form neurons of the cranial nerve nuclei belonging to special functional categories. Other specialized neuronal nuclei function as important relay points to other areas of the brain.

Myelencephalon

The myelencephalon eventually forms the medulla oblongata, a major relay center between the spinal cord and brain and a major site for autonomic regulation of vital functions such as heart rate and respiration. The larger lumen of the myelencephalon forms the fourth ventricle, and a choroid plexus develops within its roof. Developing neurons in the alar plates organize and form, lateral to medial, the somatic afferent (for cranial nerves V and VIII), special visceral afferent (for innervation of taste buds), and general visceral afferent (for interoceptive innervation of the GI tract and heart) sensory nuclei. Some alar neuroblasts also migrate ventromedially to form the olivary nuclei (major relay nuclei). The basal plates organize and form, lateral to medial, the general visceral efferent (involuntary muscles of respiration, heart, and GI tract), special visceral efferent (cranial nerves IX–XI), and somatic efferent (cranial nerve XII) motor nuclei.

Metencephalon

The alar and basal plates of the metencephalon also form important relay and cranial nerve nuclei, but the metencephalon develops 2 additional structures, the pons and cerebellum. The alar plate in this region forms 3 major sensory nuclei, the somatic afferent (contains the trigeminal neurons and portion of the vestibuloacoustic neurons), special visceral afferent, and general visceral afferent nuclei (**Part B**). The basal plate forms 3 basic motor nuclei, the general visceral efferent (supply submandibular and sublingual glands), special visceral efferent (neurons of the cranial nerves V and VII), and somatic efferent

(cranial nerve VI) nuclei. Nerve fiber tracts develop below and medial to the developing plates in an area called the *pons*. These nerve fibers relay input between the higher cortical centers of the cerebrum and cerebellum and relay input between these centers and the spinal cord. Some alar plate cells migrate ventromedially, enter the pons, and form relay nuclei called *pontine nuclei*.

The fourth ventricle of the myelencephalon extends cranially into the metencephalon. In the cranial metencephalon, the dorsal alar plate bordering the roof plate of the ventricle enlarges and begins to overlap the roof, forming *rhombic lips* (**Part B**). Meanwhile, a deep flexure (pontine flexure) develops within the pons and essentially pushes the cranial portion of the metencephalon back onto its caudal portion, thereby squashing the diamond-shaped fourth ventricle and flattening it in the cranial-caudal direction (**Parts B** and **C**). Consequently, a portion of the rhombic lips now forms a horizontal plate (cerebellar plate) overhanging the roof of the fourth ventricle. The lateral portions of the cerebellar plate enlarge and generate the cerebellar hemispheres that cover the pons, fourth ventricle, and myelencephalon; the central intervening part becomes the vermis.

Initially, the cerebellar plate consists of ventricular, mantle, and marginal layers, but eventually it is transformed into 5 layers (**Part C**). A second wave of neuroblast proliferation begins within the mantle layer adjacent to the ventricular layer. Some of these new cells form deep cerebellar nuclei like the dentate nucleus. Other cells begin migrating through the marginal layer toward the surface and establish another layer, the external granular layer. Neuroblasts within the external granular layer continue to proliferate and then differentiate into various neuron types, eventually forming the cerebellar cortex. The external granular layer gives rise to various cell layers: the innermost granular layer, the intermediate Purkinje layer, and outermost molecular layer. During the development of the cerebellar cortex, the hemispheres also undergo extensive folding, forming lobes, lobules, and gyri, and eventually they reach their definitive size sometime after birth. The cerebellum is the coordinating center for posture, movement, balance, and hearing. Its deep nuclei relay the signals while its cortex coordinates many of them.

Brain Anomalies

Cerebellar dysplasia (an abnormal number of cerebellar neurons) may or may not produce symptoms, depending on its extent. When it does, patients usually exhibit abnormal coordination of movement and speech. Cerebellar dysplasia is associated with elevated exposure to mercury; chromosomal anomalies, including trisomy 13, 18, or 21; or chromosomal deletions. Some cerebellar ataxias are caused by autosomal recessive inheritance (e.g., Friedreich's ataxia, Joubert's syndrome, and Dandy-Walker syndrome) or an X-linked recessive trait (e.g., Paine syndrome). Friedreich's syndrome accounts for one of the more common ataxias. It is characterized by a clumsy gait, ataxia of the upper limb, and slurred speech.

Nervous System III: The Midbrain and Forebrain

A. Mesencephalon

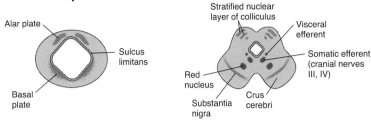

Alar plate

Sulcus limitans

Basal plate

Stratified nuclear layer of colliculus

Visceral efferent

Somatic efferent (cranial nerves III, IV)

Red nucleus

Substantia nigra

Crus cerebri

B. Ventricles of Diencephalon and Telencephalon

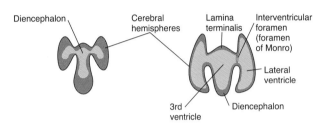

Diencephalon

Cerebral hemispheres

Lamina terminalis

Interventricular foramen (foramen of Monro)

Lateral ventricle

3rd ventricle

Diencephalon

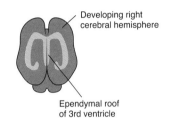

Developing right cerebral hemisphere

Ependymal roof of 3rd ventricle

C. Development of Diencephalon and Telencephalon

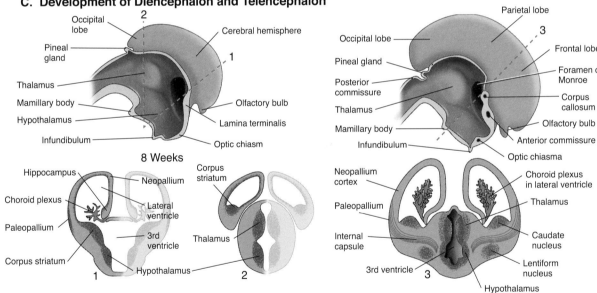

Occipital lobe

2

Cerebral hemisphere

1

Pineal gland

Thalamus

Mamillary body

Hypothalamus

Infundibulum

Olfactory bulb

Lamina terminalis

Optic chiasm

8 Weeks

Parietal lobe

3

Occipital lobe

Frontal lobe

Pineal gland

Posterior commissure

Thalamus

Mamillary body

Infundibulum

Foramen of Monroe

Corpus callosum

Olfactory bulb

Anterior commissure

Optic chiasma

Hippocampus

Neopallium

Corpus striatum

Choroid plexus

Lateral ventricle

Paleopallium

3rd ventricle

Corpus striatum

Thalamus

1

Hypothalamus

2

Neopallium cortex

Paleopallium

Internal capsule

3rd ventricle

3

Choroid plexus in lateral ventricle

Thalamus

Caudate nucleus

Lentiform nucleus

Hypothalamus

D. Development of Outer Surface of Cerebral Hemispheres

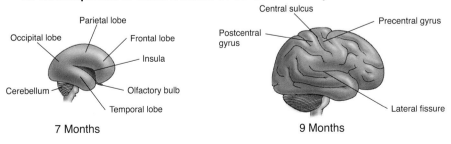

Central sulcus

Parietal lobe

Occipital lobe

Frontal lobe

Precentral gyrus

Postcentral gyrus

Insula

Cerebellum

Olfactory bulb

Temporal lobe

Lateral fissure

7 Months

9 Months

OVERVIEW

The midbrain and forebrain retain the basic alar and basal organization found in the other brain segments. In the mesencephalon, the alar plate and the basal plate generate several nuclei for the cranial nerves. The mesencephalon also develops several nuclei that serve as major relays for sensory input. The alar segment of the diencephalon makes the thalamus, hypothalamus, and posterior pituitary, whereas the basal plate has little contribution. The telencephalon forms the cerebral hemispheres and lateral ventricles. The cerebral cortex forms from proliferating ventricular neuroblasts that migrate into the outer cortex and establish several neuronal layers. Therefore, gray matter comprises the bulk of the outer cerebral hemispheres, and white matter comprises the bulk of the inner cerebrum. A vast amount of nerve fiber and synapse formation occurs during the fetal period. Therefore, the brain is very susceptible to teratogenic agents (e.g., alcohol) during the fetal period.

Mesencephalon

The mesencephalon retains the basic alar and basal organization found in the other brain segments, but the central canal narrows to form the cerebral aqueduct of Sylvius (**Part A**). Within the alar region, 2 pairs of nuclei develop. The more cranial pair forms the superior colliculi, whereas the more caudal pair forms the inferior colliculi. These nuclei serve as relays for sensory input to the cerebral cortex. The basilar plate is less well structured and generally referred to as the *tegmentum of the mesencephalon.* Within the tegmentum, basal plate neuroblasts form the motor nuclei of cranial nerve III (somatic efferent). A smaller motor nucleus also develops from the basal plate, and it innervates the papillary sphincter of the pupil. Cranial nerve IV motor nuclei within the tegmentum originate from migrating neuroblasts generated within the metencephalon. The red nuclei and substantia nigra are relay nuclei found in the tegmentum, but their origin is unclear. These nuclei primarily relay auditory and visual information between the colliculi and cerebral cortex. The marginal layer of the mesencephalon also develops bundles of fiber tracts called *peduncles* that run between and connect the cerebral cortex with the cerebellum and spinal cord.

Diencephalon

The prosencephalon generates bilateral bulges, which go on to form the telencephalon and lateral ventricles. The remaining portion of the prosencephalon connecting the telencephalon to the midbrain forms the diencephalon and the third ventricle (**Part B**). In the diencephalon, the basal plate never really organizes, and the bulk of the diencephalon originates from the alar plates. As the third ventricle enlarges within the diencephalon, it displaces the alar plates laterally. Neuroblasts within the alar plate form important relay nuclei between the cerebral hemispheres and the lower nervous system, with the dorsal-most portion forming the thalamus and the more ventral portion forming the hypothalamus (**Part C**). The thalamus is responsible for relaying all information to the cerebral cortex from the lower central nervous system, as well as auditory, visual, and olfactory information. Nuclei within the hypothalamus are principally involved in regulating homeostasis as well as regulating pituitary gland secretions.

As the third ventricle expands, it develops a midline ventral diverticulum in the floor of the diencephalon that runs toward the pharynx. This diverticulum, called the *infundibulum,* forms the posterior pituitary gland and pituitary stalk (see Chapter 25). The roof of the third ventricle develops a choroid plexus with specialized ependymal cells that produce CSF and neuropeptides. Moreover, 2 bilateral outpocketings that develop in the roof eventually join and form the pineal gland. Very early in the development of the neural tube, bilateral bulges protrude from the diencephalon to form the optic vesicles and optic stalk. These structures develop into the neural retina and optic nerves (cranial nerve II). Their development is described in Chapter 26.

Telencephalon

The forebrain develops 2 lateral bulges collectively referred to as the *telencephalon.* These bulges develop into the cerebral hemispheres and remain connected to one another at their cranial end by a median structure called the *lamina terminalis* (**Parts B** and **C**). The internal cavities of the telencephalon become the lateral ventricles. They communicate with the third ventricle through a small opening called the *interventricular foramen of Monro.* As each hemisphere enlarges, the telencephalon overgrows the diencephalon, mesencephalon, and a portion of the rhombencephalon. As each hemisphere expands, it is subdivided into the temporal, frontal, and parietal lobes by the formation of deep and prominent sulci (external clefts) (**Part D**). Smaller convoluting sulci with intervening hillocks (gyri) form on the surface of the hemispheres during the sixth and eighth months of gestation. The 2 expanding hemispheres would eventually contact each other in the midline were it not for the intervening dura mater (falx cerebri).

The thickness and organization of the hemispheres vary, and they develop recognizable nuclei and structures, including the hippocampus, corpus striatum (basal nuclei), and pallium (cortex) (**Part C**). The ventricular layer of the telencephalon generates neurons that migrate in waves toward the outer margin, forming layers of neurons with the cerebral cortex through a process resembling that found in the cerebellum. Because neuroblasts migrate into the marginal layer to form the external layers of the cortex, gray matter is on the outer surface of the cerebral cortex and white matter (cortical nerve fibers) is beneath it. Many of the nerve fibers leaving the cerebral cortex form a large fiber tract called the *internal capsule* that runs through the corpus striatum connecting the cerebral cortex with the thalamus, lower brain, and spinal cord. Commissural fibers connecting the hemispheres form the corpus callosum, anterior and posterior commissures, fornix commissure, and optic chiasma. Proper development and function of the cerebrum require establishing the appropriate synapses between neurons and subsequent myelination of their nerve fibers. A large proportion of neurite extension and synapse formation occurs during the fetal period but also continues into the neonatal period. Anterior projections from the telencephalon form the olfactory bulbs (cranial nerve I).

Brain Anomalies

Chromosomal anomalies, metabolic disorders, and maternal and fetal infections can cause mental and behavioral impairments, but the leading cause is fetal alcohol syndrome. Exposure to alcohol during this period perturbs neuron development and is thought to be the single most common cause of mental impairments (perhaps as high as 1/500 births). Maternal consumption of alcohol during the embryonic period also causes a much broader spectrum of congenital defects, including growth impairment, heart defects, NTDs, and craniofacial anomalies.

A. Spinal Nerves and Sympathetic Nervous System

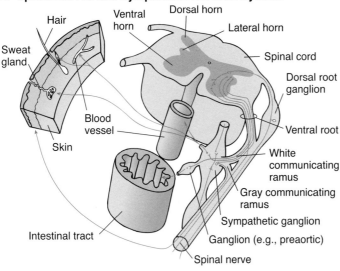

Hair

Sweat gland

Skin

Blood vessel

Intestinal tract

Ventral horn

Dorsal horn

Lateral horn

Spinal cord

Dorsal root ganglion

Ventral root

White communicating ramus

Gray communicating ramus

Sympathetic ganglion

Ganglion (e.g., preaortic)

Spinal nerve

B. Parasympathetic Nervous System

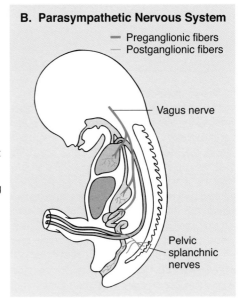

― Preganglionic fibers
― Postganglionic fibers

Vagus nerve

Pelvic splanchnic nerves

C. Suprarenal Gland

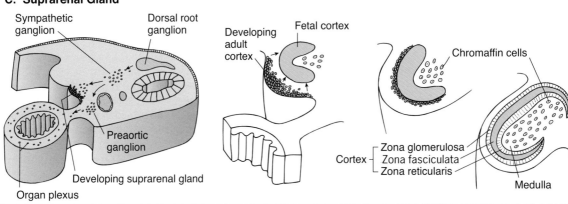

Sympathetic ganglion

Dorsal root ganglion

Preaortic ganglion

Organ plexus

Developing suprarenal gland

Developing adult cortex

Fetal cortex

Chromaffin cells

Cortex { Zona glomerulosa
Zona fasciculata
Zona reticularis

Medulla

D. Cranial Nerves

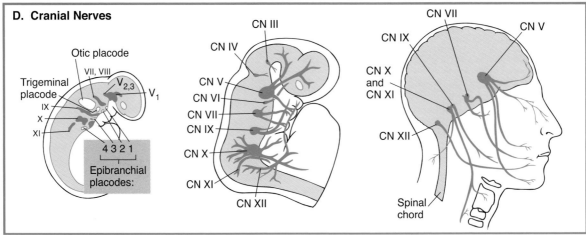

Otic placode

Trigeminal placode

VII, VIII

V2,3

V1

IX

X

XI

4 3 2 1

Epibranchial placodes:

CN III

CN IV

CN V

CN VI

CN VII

CN IX

CN X

CN XI

CN XII

CN VII

CN IX

CN X and CN XI

CN XII

CN V

Spinal chord

OVERVIEW

The peripheral nervous system consists of 2 major components: (1) the somatic component, innervating voluntary muscles and carrying cognizant sensory information, and (2) the autonomic component, innervating most of the involuntary muscles and carrying noncognizant sensory information. Somatic motor neurons develop within the spinal cord, whereas somatic sensory neurons develop outside the spinal cord. The autonomic nervous system consists of 2 divisions, the sympathetic and parasympathetic. Preganglionic sympathetic and parasympathetic neurons develop within the central nervous system. All postganglionic sympathetic and parasympathetic neurons are derived from migrating neural crest cells. Motor neurons of the cranial nerves form within the brainstem. Sensory neurons associated with the cranial nerves are derived from neural crest cells and epibranchial placodes and are located within ganglia outside the brain.

Neural Tube and Spinal Nerves

The neural tube, axial skeleton, and peripheral nerves develop in a segmental fashion along the anterior-posterior axis. The first nerves to emerge from the developing spinal cord are axons derived from ventral motor neurons. Initially, they emerge as a continuous band along the spinal cord but congregate and form discrete nerve bundles (ventral roots of the spinal nerve) (**Part A**). Meanwhile, a subset of migrating neural crest cells aggregates dorsolaterally along both sides of the neural tube in a segmental manner. These cells form the dorsal root ganglia. Sensory neuroblasts within the ganglia differentiate into unipolar neurons, with one cell process projecting into the alar plate and the other bringing back peripheral sensory information to the neuron cell body (dorsal root). The ventral and dorsal roots coalesce (distal to the dorsal root ganglia) to form a single nerve root bundle before exiting the developing vertebral canal as spinal nerves.

Sympathetics

In the thoracic region, some migrating neural crest cells localize on either side of the dorsal aorta and form the sympathetic ganglia (**Part A**). From here, some of the neural crest cells migrate into the cervical and lumbosacral levels, thereby extending the length of the sympathetic chain. Still other neural crest cells migrate ventral to the aorta and form celiac and mesenteric ganglia, and others contribute to the formation of the adrenal medulla (see below). Neurons within the lateral horn of T1–L2/L3 extend nerve processes (preganglionic fibers) that penetrate and synapse with neurons of the sympathetic ganglia. These preganglionic fibers pass from the spinal nerves into the sympathetic chain via white communicating rami. While some synapse with postganglionic sympathetic neurons at the same spinal level, others pass through and synapse in ganglia more cranial or caudal in the chain or exit to synapse with the preaortic ganglia. Axons of the sympathetic neurons (postganglionic fibers) exit the chain and re-enter the spinal nerves via the gray communicating rami to innervate most of the body. Some postganglionic fibers exit the chain and run directly into the viscera. Postganglionic fibers exiting the preaortic ganglia (e.g., the celiac and mesenteric ganglia) also directly innervate the viscera.

Parasympathetics

Parasympathetic neurons within the brainstem extend preganglionic fibers that travel within cranial nerves III, VII, IX, and X for distribution in the head and in the viscera superior to the hindgut (**Part B**). Parasympathetic neurons also develop within the lateral horn of the spinal cord at sacral levels S2–S4. Here, preganglionic fibers emerge as pelvic splanchnic nerves that enter the viscera of the hindgut and synapse with neurons in the parasympathetic ganglia of the hindgut. Parasympathetic ganglia are derived from neural crest cells and are usually located near or within the target organs and tissues (e.g., sphenopalatine, ciliary, otic, submandibular, enteric, and cardiac ganglia). Hence, the postganglionic parasympathetic fibers are usually short.

Suprarenal (Adrenal) Gland

During the fifth week, mesothelial cells between the mesenteric root of the gut and the developing gonad proliferate and penetrate the underlying mesenchyme (**Part C**). These cells differentiate into large acidophilic cells forming the fetal adrenal cortex. A second wave of mesothelial migration and proliferation occurs, forming a thinner adult cortex that nearly surrounds the entire fetal cortex. By the second postnatal month, the fetal cortex suddenly regresses except for the outermost layer, which differentiates into a recticular zone. The zona glomerulosa and zona fasciculata develop from the adult cortex during the late fetal period. The fetal adrenal cortex influences maturation of the lungs, liver, and digestive tract and may regulate parturition. The adrenal medulla develops from migrating neural crest cells adjacent to the developing fetal cortex. These cells differentiate into chromaffin cells, which are specialized postglanglionic sympathetic neurons innervated by preganglionic sympathetic fibers that release epinephrine and norepinephrine upon sympathetic stimulation.

Neurons of Cranial Nerves (Part D)

The motor neurons for the cranial nerves are located primarily within the brainstem and are discussed in previous chapters. The primary sensory neurons associated with the cranial nerves develop and reside outside the brain and project their axons into the brainstem nuclei of the alar plate. Cells comprising the sensory ganglia are derived from neural crest cells and epibranchial ectodermal placodes. Epibranchial ectodermal placodes are similar to nasal and otic placodes except they develop within the ectoderm just dorsal to the pharyngeal arches. Along with neural crest cells, epibranchial placodal cells generate neurons of the sensory ganglia of cranial nerves V, VII, IX, and X.

Anomalies

Aganglionic megacolon (Hirschsprung's disease) is the congenital absence of parasympathetic ganglia within the bowel (1/5,000 live births). The lack of peristalsis causes obstruction and enlargement of the bowel proximal to the aganglionic segment. Aganglionic segments must be resected and removed, because they are life-threatening. Congenital adrenal hyperplasia usually is caused by a genetically determined deficiency of the adrenal cortical enzymes necessary for the synthesis of particular steroids. This reduction can lead to increased ACTH secretion, causing adrenal hyperplasia of the cortex. Adrenal hyperplasia results in excessive synthesis of other androgens and during childhood accelerates skeletal maturation. It also can cause female pseudohermaphrodism (see Chapter 20).

QUESTIONS

For each of the following questions, choose the **one best answer.**

1. What structure develops from the ventral mesentery of the embryonic gut?

(A) Pancreatic islet cells

(B) Gastrosplenic ligament

(C) Greater omentum

(D) Spleen

(E) Hepatogastric ligament

2. A male newborn from a pregnancy complicated by polyhydramnios began projectile vomiting within a few hours after his first feeding. Bile was found in the vomitus. Ultrasound examination also showed that his stomach and cranial duodenum were distended. What is your diagnosis?

(A) Pyloric stenosis

(B) Duodenal atresia

(C) Malrotation of the gut

(D) Esophageal atresia

(E) Congenital hiatal hernia

3. A 5-year-old boy was examined because of a history of recurrent pain in the umbilical region. The pain was dull and burning and lasted a few days. These symptoms recurred on several occasions during the past year. Just before his visit, the boy experienced rectal bleeding and there was blood in his stool. Physical examination revealed tenderness in the anterior abdominal area in the region of the right iliac fossa. The child also showed signs of anemia. What do you suspect?

(A) Meckel's diverticulum

(B) Appendicitis

(C) Pyloric stenosis

(D) Annular pancreas

(E) Duodenal atresia

4. A near-term stillborn infant had a light gray shiny mass protruding from the umbilicus. This mass appeared to be covered by a thin transparent membrane. Autopsy results showed the mass to consist primarily of intestinal loops. What is your diagnosis?

(A) A volvulus

(B) Gastroschisis

(C) Meckel's diverticulum

(D) Persistent vitelline duct

(E) Omphalocele

Questions 5 and 6.
While examining a 6-year-old female child, the physician discovered that the child did not have a right kidney.

5. What is this condition?

(A) Bilateral renal agenesis

(B) Unilateral renal agenesis

(C) A pelvic kidney

(D) Polycystic kidney disease

(E) A horseshoe kidney

6. How might this condition be explained embryologically?

(A) The pronephric kidney on the right side degenerated.

(B) The right mesonephric kidney did not develop Bowman's capsules.

(C) Tissue-tissue interactions between the right uteric bud and metanephric mesodermal cap were abnormal.

(D) The mesonephric tubules did not produce primary nephrons.

(E) The right kidney atrophied because of numerous cysts within the early kidney.

7. Differentiation of the male gonads and ducts is dependent on a cascade of hormones and growth factors driven by the Y chromosome. Which of the following best describes this cascade in normal males?

(A) TDF → Sertoli cells → MIS → paramesonephric tubule regression

(B) TDF → Leydig cells → testosterone → paramesonephric tubule regression

(C) TDF → Sertoli cells → testosterone → paramesonephric tubule regression

(D) MIS → mesonephric tubule regression → male external genitalia development

(E) MIS → Leydig cells → mesonephric tubule retention → vas deferens development

Questions 8 and 9.
You examine a 16-year-old boy and find that his urethra opens on the ventral surface of the penis approximately 1.5 cm proximal to the glans. The opening also extends posteriorly for approximately 2 cm.

8. What is this condition?

(A) Epispadias

(B) Hypospadias

(C) Cryptorchism

(D) Patent urachus

(E) Penile urethral patency

9. What is the most likely cause?

(A) Failure of labioscrotal swellings to fuse

(B) Hypoplasia of the urethral plate

(C) Failure of urogenital folds to fuse

(D) Failure of genital tubercle to elongate

(E) Failure of the allantois to degenerate

10. A young female patient in her mid-teens visits your office complaining of periodic intense abdominal cramping that usually subsides within about a week. Upon questioning her further, you find that she has never menstruated. Physical examination showed that she had well-developed female secondary sexual characteristics, including breast development, pubic hair, and broadening of the pelvis. While a pelvic examination showed normal external genitalia, only the urethral opening was found. What is your diagnosis?

(A) A unicornate uterus

(B) A bicornate uterus

(C) Missing ovaries

(D) Uterine agenesis

(E) Vaginal agenesis

11. A mid-teen female patient visits your office wondering why, unlike her female peers, she has not had a menstrual period. Physical examination revealed a very normal female phenotype. Hypothalamic and pituitary hormone levels looked normal, but tests revealed high levels of testosterone. Moreover, her karyotype is 46, XY. What is your diagnosis?

(A) Congenital adrenal hyperplasia

(B) Female pseudohermaphrodism

(C) Klinefelter's syndrome

(D) Testicular feminization

(E) Inactive Barr body

Questions 12 and 13.
A mother was bathing her 4-month-old baby boy. As she bathed him, she noticed that his left testis was not in the scrotum. Examination by the pediatrician showed that the right side was normal and confirmed that the left testis was not in the scrotum. Further palpitation revealed a small ovoid swell in the left inguinal canal.

12. What is your diagnosis?

(A) Patent vaginal process

(B) Hydrocele

(C) Congenital inguinal hernia

(D) Gubernacular agenesis

(E) Cryptorchidism

13. How would you treat this baby?

(A) Do nothing at this time but re-examine him again in 6–8 months.

(B) Surgically place the testis into the scrotum.

(C) Treat the baby with testosterone.

(D) Treat the baby with corticosteroids.

(E) Treat the left cremasteric muscle with a small dose of α-bungarotoxin.

14. A 4-year-old girl was still in diapers because she continually wet them. Ultrasound examination showed 2 normal-appearing kidneys, but a urogram detected only a right ureter and right kidney. Upon closer pelvic examination, the physician noticed that urine was coming from the vagina as well as the presence of a small opening in the left posterior vaginal wall. What is the most likely diagnosis?

(A) Rectovaginal fistula

(B) Patent urachus

(C) Ectopic ureter opening

(D) Vesiculorectal fistula

(E) Gartner's cyst

15. As a medical student, you are asked to examine the most recent arrival in the neonatal ward. You observe that the right hand is missing the fourth and fifth digits and that the second and third digits are fused. What term would you use to describe the anomaly of the second and third digits?

(A) Syndactyly

(B) Brachydactyly

(C) Polydactyly

(D) Adactyly

(E) Phocomelia

16. A baby missing the entire upper right limb was delivered. What could be one possible explanation for this congenital defect?

(A) Myotomal cells from the corresponding somites did not enter the upper right limb bud.

(B) The apical epidermal ridge did not develop on the right upper limb bud.

(C) Segmental spinal nerves did not enter the upper right limb bud.

(D) There was excessive apoptosis (cell death) within the digital plate of the right limb bud.

(E) The lateral plate mesoderm did not differentiate into chondrocytes within the limb bud.

17. An infant has a long wedge-shaped skull and you are asked for your opinion regarding a diagnosis. Closer examination reveals that the sutures between the parietal bones prematurely fused. What would be your initial diagnosis?

(A) Hydrocephaly

(B) Achondrogenesis

(C) Scaphocephaly

(D) Oxycephaly

(E) Stenosis of the cerebral aqueduct of Sylvius

18. Which of the following bones is derived from neural crest cells found within the second pharyngeal arch?

(A) Mandible

(B) Greater horn of the hyoid bone

(C) Malleus

(D) Stapes

(E) Greater wing of the sphenoid bone

19. A newborn is delivered with a cleft lip. What structures did not properly fuse?

(A) Medial nasal process and lateral nasal process

(B) Medial nasal process and maxillary process

(C) Lateral nasal process and maxillary process

(D) Mandibular process and maxillary process

(E) Lateral nasal process and frontonasal process

20. A pediatrician examined a newborn in the neonatal unit because of difficulty in feeding. The baby eagerly accepted the milk placed in the mouth with a dropper but had difficulty in suckling when a nipple was used. What congenital anomaly could be responsible for this?

(A) First arch syndrome

(B) Abnormal innervation of cranial nerve IX

(C) Pierre Robin syndrome

(D) Median cleft in the hard palate

(E) Treacher Collins syndrome

Questions 21 and 22.
A 20-year-old female patient has a noticeable swelling in her neck that recently began increasing in size. The swelling was located beneath the anterior border of the sternocleidomastoid muscle, about two thirds up from its clavicular origin.

21. What is your initial diagnosis?

(A) Thyroglossal cyst

(B) Cervical cyst

(C) Accessory thyroid tissue

(D) Accessory tonsils

(E) Atresia of the internal acoustical meatus

22. What could be the embryological origin of this swelling?

(A) The first pharyngeal groove

(B) The second pharyngeal pouch

(C) The thyroglossal duct

(D) The second and third pharyngeal pouches

(E) The cervical sinus

23. A pregnant mother had a bad bout with rubella during the fifth and sixth weeks of her pregnancy. What is one possible consequence of this infection?

(A) There is an increased risk that the baby will have congenital cataracts.

(B) There is an increased risk that the baby will have coloboma of the iris.

(C) There is an increased risk that the baby will have microagnathia.

(D) There is an increased risk that the baby will have anotia.

(E) There is no increased risk of congenital anomalies.

Questions 24 and 25.
In a conversation with a new acquaintance, you notice that this person is missing a small area of the lower right iris.

24. What is this condition?

(A) Cryptophthalmos

(B) Microphthalmia

(C) Anophthalmia

(D) Hyaloid artery degeneration

(E) Coloboma of the iris

25. What causes it?

(A) Failure of choroid fissure to close

(B) Abnormal neural crest migration

(C) Abnormal interactions between the optic vesicle and ectoderm

(D) Posterior chamber cavitation

(E) Weak adhesion between the inner and outer layers of the optic vesicle

26. A young man goes to his physician to complain about a swelling in his neck just below the hyoid bone. What might this swelling be?

(A) An accessory thymus

(B) A cervical cyst

(C) A thyroglossal cyst

(D) An aberrant ultimobranchial body

(E) A tracheoesophageal fistula

Questions 27 and 28.
A 2-year-old was taken to a pediatrician because the mother suspected deafness in the right ear. The left ear was found to be normal, but examination of the right ear revealed that the external auditory meatus ended blindly about a centimeter from the exterior surface. The child could hear the vibration of a tuning fork when placed on the right mastoid process.

27. What is your diagnosis?

(A) Congenital absence of the spiral ganglia

(B) Anotia

(C) Microtia

(D) Congenital absence of the hair cells

(E) Congenital atresia of the external auditory meatus

28. What is the normal embryological origin of this structure?

(A) Pharyngeal groove 1

(B) Pharyngeal arch 2

(C) The otic placode

(D) Pharyngeal pouch 1

(E) Special visceral afferent neurons from the alar plate of the metencephalon

29. Which of the following is the correct temporal sequence for the histogenesis and differentiation of cell types and layers derived from the neuroepithelium of the neural tube?

(A) Neuroepithelial cells → ventricular layer → mantle layer → marginal layer

(B) Neuroepithelial cells → glioblasts → ependymal cells → astrocytes

(C) Neuroepithelial cells → neuroblasts → glioblasts → microglia

(D) Neuroepithelial cells → glioblasts → oligodendrocytes → microglia

(E) Neuroepithelial cells → marginal layer → mantle layer → ventricular layer

30. A 4-month-old boy was taken to his pediatrician because his mother noticed that his head seemed larger than normal and she thought that it was slowly getting bigger. Physical examination showed that the anterior and posterior fontanelles were too large for the size of his face, and neurological examination showed signs of optic atrophy and increased muscle tone within the limbs. What is your diagnosis?

(A) Craniosynostosis

(B) Hydrocephaly

(C) Cranial meningomyelocele

(D) Oxycephaly

(E) Accelerated chondrogenesis of the calvaria

31. The cell bodies of the spinal nerve motor neurons arise in what structure(s)?

(A) Alar plates

(B) Basal plates

(C) Lateral horns

(D) Roof plate

(E) Dorsal root ganglia

32. You examined a young boy with clumsy gait and ataxia of the arms. While taking his history, you noticed that he slurred many of his words. His family history also indicated that he might have inherited this disorder as an autosomal recessive trait. What is your initial diagnosis?

(A) Cri du chat syndrome

(B) Huntington's chorea

(C) Fetal alcohol syndrome

(D) Arnold-Chiari malformation

(E) Friedreich's syndrome

33. Which of the following structures is *not* derived from the diencephalon?

(A) Thalamus

(B) Pineal gland

(C) Cerebrum

(D) Hypothalamus

(E) Optic vesicle

34. What is responsible for pushing the developing cerebellum back over and dorsal to the fourth ventricle?

(A) Formation of the pontine flexure

(B) Expansion of the myelencephalon roof plate

(C) Formation of the mesencephalic flexure

(D) Formation of the cervical flexure

(E) Expansion of the telencephalon

35. As a child psychiatrist, you tested an 8-year-old girl and found that she has mental impairments. No other congenital anomalies were apparent, but medical records show that she exhibited signs of intrauterine growth restriction as a newborn. Extensive genetic testing revealed no chromosomal anomalies and no familial history of mental impairments. What explanation may account for the mental impairment?

(A) The mother had a deficiency in folic acid during the gestational period.

(B) The child was exposed to alcohol during the fetal period.

(C) The child was exposed to alcohol during the embryonic period.

(D) The child was exposed to rubella virus during the embryonic period.

(E) The mother had diabetes mellitus.

36. A 2-day-old baby in the neonatal ward began vomiting meconium and had a distended abdomen. The baby also had a number of non-pigmented patches of skin. Radiograms showed a large expanded segment of colon above a more distal constricted segment. What is your initial diagnosis?

(A) Annular pancreas

(B) Hirschsprung's disease

(C) Pyloric stenosis

(D) Meckel's diverticulum

(E) Rectal atresia

37. Which of the following neural elements would be derived from epibranchial placodes?

(A) Preganglionic sympathetic neurons

(B) Motor neurons of cranial nerves

(C) Sensory neurons of cranial nerves

(D) Motor neurons of the ventral horns

(E) Glia in the dorsal root ganglia

ANSWERS

1. The answer is E.

The hepatogastric ligament is derived from the caudal border of the ventral mesentery (the lesser omentum), and it stretches between the liver and the stomach. The gastrosplenic ligament and greater omentum as well as the nonhematopoietic elements of the spleen are derived from the dorsal mesentery. Pancreatic islet cells are likely derived from the endoderm of the pancreatic buds.

2. The answer is B.

Duodenal atresia is an obstruction of the duodenum usually caused by incomplete recanalization of the duodenal lumen. In this case, the obstruction was below the entrance of the bile duct, as suggested by the presence of bile in the vomitus. Moreover, the stomach and duodenal segment cranial to the obstruction became distended, and feeding exacerbated the problem, leading to vomiting. An annular pancreas can also produce similar symptoms. This obstruction also prevented passage and uptake of amniotic fluid by the fetus and was likely the cause of the polyhydramniotic condition observed during pregnancy. Duodenal atresia must be corrected surgically.

3. The answer is A.

Meckel's diverticulum is found in 2%–4% of the population but is more prevalent in males than females. An ileal diverticulum (Meckel's) can become inflamed and can present symptoms similar to appendicitis. The wall of the diverticulum contains all the same tissue layers as found in the rest of the ileum, but it may also contain patches of gastric or pancreatic tissue. In this case, gastric mucosal tissue was present and secreted acid, resulting in a bleeding ulcer, umbilical tenderness, and a bloody stool. After treatment of the anemia, surgery would likely be performed to excise the diverticulum and reanastomose the ileum.

4. The answer is E.

Omphalocele is an anomaly whereby the intestinal loops from the physiological hernia do not completely return into the abdominal cavity. The thin membrane covering the omphalocele consists of the parietal peritoneum and amnion. The prognosis is not very good as almost 25% of these individuals die before birth, and anywhere between 50% and 80% of these individuals have other anomalies. If born alive and the omphalocele is the only defect, the infant has a good chance of surviving with surgical repair. With gastroschisis, the intestines herniate outside the abdomen because the abdominal walls fail to close. In that situation, the herniated viscera are exposed to the amniotic fluid in utero and the outside air after birth.

5 and 6. The answers are B and C, respectively.

This child has only 1 kidney because the right kidney did not develop (unilateral renal agenesis). The most likely cause of this condition was aberrant tissue-tissue interactions between the right ureteric bud and the adjacent metanephric cap mesoderm. This interaction is required for continual branching of the ureteric bud. The ureteric bud is responsible for generating the collecting tubules and ducts, renal pelvis, and ureters of the adult kidney. This tissue-tissue interaction also drives the formation of Bowman's capsule, proximal and distal convoluted tubules, and loop of Henle from the metanephric cap mesoderm. The

glomerulus and renal blood vessels develop from the urogenital ridge mesoderm. Having 1 normal-functioning kidney is asymptomatic.

7. The answer is A.

TDF is on the Y chromosome and is responsible for generating Sertoli cells from the primary sex cords. Together with primordial germ cells, the Sertoli cells form the seminiferous tubules. Sertoli cells produce MIS, which represses development of the paramesonephric tubule. TDF is also responsible for the differentiation of Leydig cells from interstitial mesodermal cells. Testosterone from Leydig cells promotes mesonephric development and the male duct system. Testosterone is also converted into dihydrotestosterone by 5α-hydroxylase, and dihydrotestosterone is the substance primarily responsible for driving male external genital development.

8 and 9. The answers are B and C, respectively.

Hypospadias is the condition whereby the penile urethra opens anywhere along the ventral side of the penis. It is the most common malformation of the penis. The opening can vary in size from very small to elongated and cleftlike running almost the entire length of the penis. It is usually caused by an incomplete fusion of the urogenital folds, which develop on both sides of the urogenital plate. The glans portion of the penile urethra develops from an ectodermal ingrowth extending in from the tip of the glans to the urethral plate. This ingrowth canalizes, connecting the external penile meatus of the glans to the rest of the penile urethra.

10. The answer is E.

Vaginal agenesis usually occurs as a consequence of failed vaginal plate development. Interactions between the fused paramesonephric ducts and the urogenital sinus stimulate an endodermal ingrowth called the vaginal (sinovaginal) plate. This plate elongates and canalizes, forming the vagina and the lower uterus. The upper portion of the uterus and uterine horns are derived from the paramesonephric tubules. Although the vagina and lower uterus are missing, in this case the paramesonephric portion of the uterus still developed and underwent endometrial changes associated with the teenager's menstrual cycle. But with the vaginal agenesis, the menstrual flow was curtailed, causing the intense abdominal cramping, pain, and inflammation. Eventually the inflammation and pain subsided but reappeared with the next menstrual cycle.

11. The answer is D.

This is a case of male pseudohermaphrodism where the karyotype and gonads are male but the external phenotype is female. While inadequate steroidal synthesis can lead to feminization of the external genitalia, tests showed normal levels of hypothalamic and pituitary hormones. Therefore, the most likely explanation is androgen insensitivity syndrome (testicular feminization) whereby the individual's testosterone receptors are not functional. Leydig cells within the testis secrete testosterone. The testosterone levels were elevated because of reduced testosterone-dependent negative feedback. Without the influence of testosterone, the external genitalia developed along the female phenotype. Secondary female characteristics including breast enlargement and pelvic widening subsequently developed because of the influence of normally produced male estrogens that were not masked by the testosterone.

12 and 13. **The answers are E and A, respectively.**

Cryptorchism is an undescended testis and is common. A cryptorchid testis can be found within the abdomen or anywhere along the route of the gubernaculum. A cryptorchid testis will usually complete its descent within the first year on its own. Therefore, it is advisable to do nothing during the first year or two but to closely monitor the situation. If the testis does not descend into the scrotum by the time the infant reaches age 4–5 years, then surgery is recommended. If the testis is left in the abdomen or inguinal canal, the higher body temperature in these areas can cause irreversible damage to the seminiferous tubules. Moreover, about 50% of affected individuals with an undescended testis eventually develop testicular metastasis.

14. **The answer is C.**

The developing ureters are derived from ureteric buds that grow out from the urogenital sinus (future bladder) into the metanephric mesoderm. Differential growth is responsible for the posterior positioning of the ureter openings in the bladder. In females, the vagina develops from an endodermal outgrowth of the urogenital sinus (the vaginal plate) near this same area. This rod of endoderm eventually canalizes, forming the vagina and lower uterus. Because of the developing vagina's close proximity to the ureter openings, the ureters may open into the vagina rather than the urogenital sinus (bladder). In this patient, only the left ureteric opening was ectopic (i.e., opening into the vagina). Surgery connecting the ureter to the bladder will remedy this situation.

15. **The answer is A.**

When 2 or more digits are fused, it is called syndactyly. Fusion may be at the level of the soft tissues, like webbed fingers, or extend to the level of the bone. Webbed fingers are likely due to insufficient cell death (apoptosis), which is necessary for separating the soft tissues of the digits. In contrast, fusion at the bone level is more likely due to an abnormal number of mesodermal condensations generated within the digital plate responsible for producing the cartilage and bone. Brachydactyly is the term used for abnormally short digits, while polydactyly is the term used to describe the presence of extra digits. Adactyly is the term used to describe the congenital absence of digits.

16. **The answer is B.**

The apical epidermal ridge found at the tip of the newly formed limb bud is essential for limb development. It is primarily responsible for the continued extension and growth of the limb bud. If it does not form, regresses, or is removed, the limb will not form, leading to amelia.

17. **The answer is C.**

Craniosynostosis is a congenital defect due to premature closure of the cranial sutures that results in abnormal development of the cranium. Scaphocephaly results if the parietal sutures close prematurely, causing the skull to take on a long, narrow, and wedge-shaped appearance as seen in this case. Oxycephaly involves premature closure of the coronal or lamboid suture, producing a tower-like skull. The most severe forms of craniosynostosis occur if premature closure occurs while in utero. Craniosynostosis can lead to increases in CSF pressure that if severe enough, can cause mental impairment.

18. **The answer is D.**

Neural crest cells in the second pharyngeal arch generate Reichert's cartilage. This cartilage forms the primordia for the stapes, styloid process, stylohyoid ligament, and the lesser horns and upper rim of the hyoid bone. Neural crest–derived mesenchymal cells in the first pharyngeal arch generate the maxilla, mandible, malleus and incus, greater wing of the sphenoid bone, and parts of the zygomatic, sphenoid, and temporal bones. Unlike the bones in the first arch (the exception being the malleus and incus), bones in the second and third arches form through endochondrial bone formation.

19. **The answer is B.**

The medial nasal processes adjacent to each nasal pit eventually meet in the midline to form the intermaxillary process. The external part of the intermaxillary process forms the philtrum. The intermaxillary process then fuses with each maxillary process, and together they make the entire upper lip. If fusion between the exterior portion of the intramaxillary process (fused medial nasal processes) and maxillary process fails on one side of the face, the result is a unilateral cleft lip. If it fails on both sides, the result is a bilateral cleft lip.

20. **The answer is D.**

The physician discovered the baby had a median cleft palate that was not accompanied by a cleft lip. The difficulty in feeding stemmed from the absence of an intact palate, making it difficult for the infant to suckle. Yet, if milk was placed in the mouth with a dropper, the baby could feed. Therefore, the swallowing response was intact. With this condition, the baby could continue to feed in this manner, but care must be taken not to let milk aspirate into the nasal cavity. This can increase the risk of pneumonia and choking. Surgical repair should be undertaken as soon as possible and before the child begins speaking.

21 and 22. **The answers are B and E, respectively.**

The second pharyngeal arch overgrows and covers the second, third, and fourth pharyngeal grooves, forming a transient cervical sinus. Normally this sinus regresses; however, if it does not, a lateral cervical (branchial) cyst will form. This cyst may remain unnoticed for an entire lifetime, but at anytime it can begin to increase in size. Lateral cervical cysts can become infected and should be surgically removed. Occasionally, these cysts open to the exterior, forming a cervical (branchial) fistula, and small amounts of mucus secreted by the epithelial lining of the cyst can be extruded onto the surface of the neck.

23. **The answer is A.**

Rubella infections can lead to congenital cataracts, glaucoma, and deafness (targeting development of the organ of Corti). There is also an increased risk that the baby will have a patent ductus arteriosus.

24 and 25. **The answers are E and A, respectively.**

During early development of the optic vesicle, a groove called the choroid fissure develops in the lower part of the optic cup and optic stalk. This fissure houses the developing hyaloid artery, and as the fissure closes, it envelops the hyaloid artery. However, if the fissure does not completely close, iris formation in the lower part of the eye cannot occur. This is referred to as coloboma of the iris. Individuals with this anomaly may be more sensitive to bright light because the pupil cannot be closed in this region. While neural crest cells provide cells making the stroma and pupillary muscles of the iris, these cells migrate into the iris after its initial formation. Therefore, abnormal migration and differentiation of neural crest cells are not responsible for the gap. Anophthalmia is the absence of eyes, whereas microphthalmia is small or tiny eyes. These two defects are likely due to abnormal interactions between the ectoderm and optic vesicles.

26. The answer is C.

This is most likely a thyroglossal cyst arising from a remnant of the thyroglossal duct. This duct develops during thyroid gland development and usually degenerates. However, if remnants persist, they can form cysts. These cysts can develop anywhere along the pathway taken by the descending thyroid primordium (i.e., running from the foramen cecum of the tongue to below the anterior larynx where it normally resides in a newborn). Thyroglossal cysts, when they do occur, frequently develop just below the hyoid bone. These cysts do not contain thyroid tissue. However, accessory thyroid tissue sometimes can be found along this same route and is subject to the same regulatory and pathological conditions as normal glandular tissue.

27 and 28. The answers are E and A, respectively.

The external acoustic meatus develops from a solid core of ectoderm growing medially from the base of the first pharyngeal groove. This solid ectodermal core eventually canalizes, forming the external auditory meatus. In this patient, either the ectodermal core did not develop, or if it did, it never canalized. The right inner ear was intact, as this child could hear vibrations generated by a tuning fork placed on the right mastoid process.

29. The answer is A.

The early neural tube consists only of neuroepithelial cells. The cell bodies of dividing neuroepithelial cells move toward the luminal side of the neural tube, forming a layer called the ventricular layer. As the cells continue to proliferate, the daughter cells (neuroblasts) aggregate into another layer called the mantle layer, just peripheral to the ventricular layer. The developing neurons in the mantle layer begin extending neurites up and down the neural tube in a layer just peripheral to the mantle layer. This forms the third layer, the marginal layer. The neuroepithelial cells first generate neuroblasts (the progenitors for neurons) but then begin producing glial stem cells called glioblasts. The glioblasts divide and differentiate into astrocytes and oligodendrocytes. Lastly, neuroepithelial cells begin producing ependymal cells. These cells line the ventricles of the brain and lumen of the spinal cord. Microglia are not derived from the neuroepithelium; rather they are derived from mesodermal cells that take up residence within the central nervous system where they function much like macrophages.

30. The answer is B.

Given there were no other known anomalies, the most likely cause of the hydrocephaly was a stenosis or blockage of the cerebral aqueduct (of Sylvius). Because the choroid plexus continually produces CSF, CSF must pass through the cerebral aqueduct to gain access to the brain surface and sagittal sinus where it can be resorbed. When unable to pass through this aqueduct, it accumulates within the lateral and third ventricles, causing the brain to swell. The fetal and newborn skull can expand because of the open cranial sutures and the presence of fontanelles. Therefore, the cranial vault increases in size in an attempt to accommodate the enlarging brain. If brain expansion exceeds the capacity of the cranial vault, intracranial pressure increases and neurological deficits ensue. In this patient, the increase in muscle tone was likely due to compression of corticospinal tracts caused by the expanding lateral ventricles, while the optic atrophy was likely due to compression of the optic nerves.

31. The answer is B.

Aggregates of neuroblasts in the basal plate differentiate into the spinal nerve motor neurons, while neuroblasts in the lateral horn (found only in axial levels T1–L2/3 and levels S2–S4) form preganglionic sympathetic and parasympathetic neurons. The alar plates form interneurons that receive and transmit sensory information provided by dorsal root ganglion neurons.

32. The answer is E.

Friedreich's syndrome is one of the more common causes of ataxia and is inherited as an autosomal recessive trait. Individuals with this syndrome exhibit the symptoms described in this patient. Cri du chat is due to a microdeletion of the short arm of chromosome 5. This disorder also manifests cerebellar deficits but is usually accompanied by other anomalies such as microcephaly, congenital heart disease, impaired intelligence, and a catlike cry.

33. The answer is C.

The cerebrum develops from the telencephalon. All the other structures listed are derived from the diencephalonic portion of the forebrain.

34. The answer is A.

As the cerebellar hemispheres begin to enlarge, a deep, dorsal flexion develops at the level of the pons (pontine flexure) in the metencephalon. This deep flexion carries the developing cerebellar hemispheres backward so they drape over the fourth ventricle and the myelencephalon. As the cerebellar hemispheres continue to expand and develop, they completely cover the myelencephalon.

35. The answer is B.

Exposure to alcohol during the fetal period primarily affects the maturation of organs and impairs fetal growth. The primary organ undergoing significant development during the fetal period is the brain. During this period, a significant amount of neuronal proliferation, neurite extension, and synapse formation is ongoing within the brain. Exposure to alcohol during this period perturbs these events. Exposure to ethanol during the embryonic period causes a much broader spectrum of congenital defects, including heart defects, NTDs, craniofacial anomalies, and others. Ethanol consumption during pregnancy is thought to be the single most common cause of mental impairment, with a frequency of occurrence thought to be as high as 1/500 births.

36. The answer is B.

The constriction of the bowel is due to congenital aganglionic megacolon (Hirschsprung's disease) whereby a segment of gut is paralyzed in a constricted state because it is missing the parasympathetic ganglia. Because of the paralysis, the part of the intestine proximal (cranial) to the aganglionic portion becomes distended as meconium and other substances accumulate. The presence of meconium in the vomitus suggests the blockage is within the large intestine. In about 75% of cases of Hirschsprung's disease, the aganglionic segment occurs within the rectosigmoidal colon. Symptoms usually show up within 48 hours. Aganglionic megacolon is due to defective colonization of the gut by neural crest cells, which are responsible for forming the parasympathetic ganglia. Other associated defects that may accompany congenital aganglionic megacolon include hypopigmentation of skin, mandibular defects, facial clefts, and pulmonary trunk defects, structures whose normal development also includes a neural crest component.

37. The answer is C.

Epibranchial placodes contribute to the generation of cranial nerve sensory neurons. Epibranchial placodes are ectodermal thickenings that form above the pharyngeal arches. These placodes generate migrating neuroblasts that together with neural crest cells produce the sensory neurons of cranial nerves V, VII, IX, and X. However, the glia of these sensory neurons are derived from neural crest cells. Ventral motor neurons develop from neuroblasts within the basal plate of the neural tube. Preganglionic sympathetic neurons develop from neuroblast aggregates within the lateral walls of the neural tube at spinal levels T1–L2/3 (the lateral horn). Sensory neurons and glial cells of the dorsal root ganglia are derived from neural crest cells.

PART III

Heart I: The Early Phase

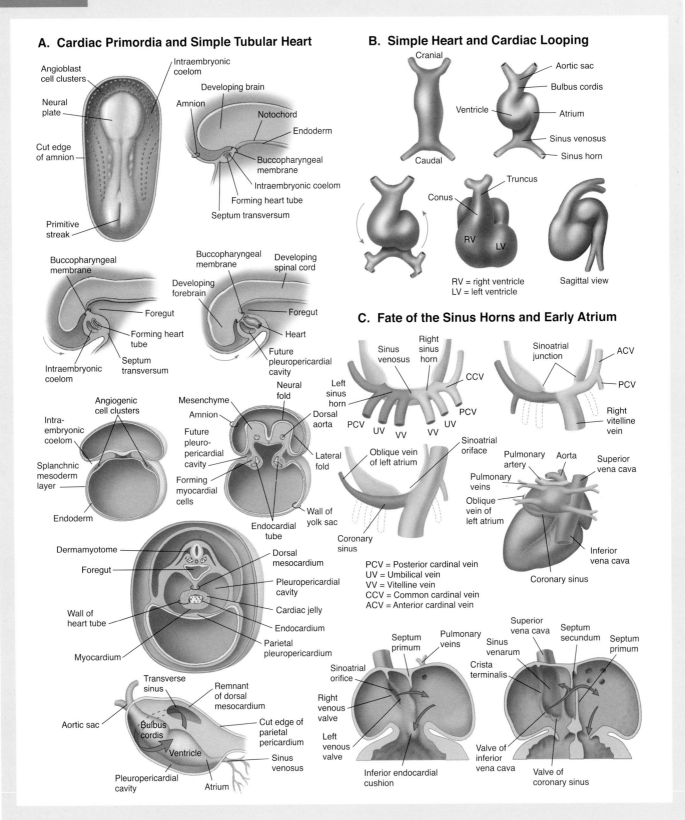

A. Cardiac Primordia and Simple Tubular Heart

Angioblast cell clusters
Intraembryonic coelom
Neural plate
Developing brain
Amnion
Notochord
Cut edge of amnion
Endoderm
Buccopharyngeal membrane
Intraembryonic coelom
Forming heart tube
Septum transversum
Primitive streak

Buccopharyngeal membrane
Buccopharyngeal membrane
Developing spinal cord
Developing forebrain
Foregut
Foregut
Forming heart tube
Heart
Intraembryonic coelom
Septum transversum
Future pleuropericardial cavity

Angiogenic cell clusters
Mesenchyme
Neural fold
Intra-embryonic coelom
Amnion
Dorsal aorta
Future pleuro-pericardial cavity
Splanchnic mesoderm layer
Lateral fold
Forming myocardial cells
Endoderm
Endocardial tube
Wall of yolk sac

Dermamyotome
Dorsal mesocardium
Foregut
Pleuropericardial cavity
Cardiac jelly
Wall of heart tube
Endocardium
Myocardium
Parietal pleuropericardium

Transverse sinus
Remnant of dorsal mesocardium
Aortic sac
Bulbus cordis
Cut edge of parietal pericardium
Ventricle
Sinus venosus
Pleuropericardial cavity
Atrium

B. Simple Heart and Cardiac Looping

Cranial
Aortic sac
Bulbus cordis
Ventricle
Atrium
Sinus venosus
Sinus horn
Caudal

Truncus
Conus
RV
LV

RV = right ventricle
LV = left ventricle
Sagittal view

C. Fate of the Sinus Horns and Early Atrium

Sinus venosus
Right sinus horn
Sinoatrial junction
ACV
CCV
PCV
Left sinus horn
Right vitelline vein
PCV
PCV
UV
VV
VV
UV

Oblique vein of left atrium
Sinoatrial oriface
Pulmonary artery
Aorta
Superior vena cava
Pulmonary veins
Oblique vein of left atrium
Coronary sinus
Inferior vena cava
Coronary sinus

PCV = Posterior cardinal vein
UV = Umbilical vein
VV = Vitelline vein
CCV = Common cardinal vein
ACV = Anterior cardinal vein

Septum primum
Pulmonary veins
Superior vena cava
Septum secundum
Sinus venarum
Septum primum
Sinoatrial orifice
Crista terminalis
Right venous valve
Left venous valve
Valve of inferior vena cava
Inferior endocardial cushion
Valve of coronary sinus

OVERVIEW

Cardiac defects are the most common life-threatening congenital defects, accounting for up to 20% of all congenital anomalies (about 1:5–8/1000 live births). The heart is the first functioning organ in the embryo. The early cardiac tube forms from splanchnic mesoderm and develops distinct segments that constitute the progenitors of the adult chambers as well as the roots of the aorta and pulmonary artery. During this early period, the tubular heart undergoes looping in order to place the primitive chambers into their adult anatomical positions. In addition, venous return to the primitive atrium is shifted to the right side before atrial septation, through differential growth and changes in hemodynamics brought about by venous anastomoses and left-to-right shunting of the systemic venous return.

Cardiac Primordia and Simple Tubular Heart

Embryonic development of the heart is mostly completed by the end of the second month. It begins with the differentiation and formation of cell clusters called angioblasts within the precardiac splanchnic mesoderm (**Part A**). Initially, this mesoderm lies under the intraembryonic coelom running cranial to the buccopharyngeal membrane and along both sides of the anterior third of the embryo. However, the precardiac mesoderm swings behind the buccopharyngeal membrane and beneath the foregut during the process of embryonic body folding. This reverses the position of the cardiogenic area so that it now lies dorsal to the intraembryonic coelom. Simultaneously, the cardiogenic angioblasts within the precardiac mesoderm coalesce to form 2 primitive endocardial tubes on either side of the developing foregut. These primitive tubes fuse to form a single midline endocardial tube during the infolding of the lateral body wall. The adjacent splanchnic mesoderm differentiates into cardiomyocytes, and extracellular matrix is deposited between the endocardium and myocardium (the cardiac jelly). This single heart tube then sinks into the underlying future pleuropericardial cavity but remains attached to the dorsal body wall by a thin layer of mesoderm, the dorsal mesocardium. The dorsal mesocardium soon ruptures in the middle, forming the future transverse sinus of the pericardial sac. Residual cells from the caudal portion of the dorsal mesocardium subsequently migrate onto the surface of the myocardium, forming the epicardium (visceral pericardium) and eventually the coronary vasculature. As the embryo continues to grow, cranial flexion carries the primitive developing heart into the cervical and then the thoracic region, pulling the cranial portion of the connected dorsal aorta along with it. This process forms the first aortic arch. Eventually 4 additional pairs of intervening aortic arches will connect the outflow portion of the heart to the paired dorsal aortae. Meanwhile, continued vasculogenesis and angiogenesis connect the caudal end of the heart with 3 pairs of vessels, the common cardinal veins, vitelline veins, and umbilical veins.

The simple tubular heart develops a series of constrictions and expansions, dividing it into regions (**Part B**). The cardiac regions in the direction of venous-to-arterial blood flow are the sinus venosus, primitive atrium, atrioventricular region, primitive ventricle, bulbus cordis, and aortic sac. The sinus venosus is the confluens of the right and left sinus horns, and each horn collects blood from the umbilical, vitelline, and common cardinal veins. The sinus venosus then empties into the primitive atrium, where blood is propelled through the atrioventricular canal into the primitive ventricle. The primitive ventricle is the precursor to the adult left ventricle and is delineated from the bulbus cordis by a constriction called the bulboventricular sulcus. The bulbus cordis will subdivide further into the right ventricle, conus arteriosus, and truncus arteriosus. The aortic sac is located at the cranial-most end of the bulbus cordis and serves as the common outlet for the aortic arch arteries. The aortic sac and truncus arteriosus eventually divide to form the aorta, pulmonary artery, and roots of the great arteries. Once the single tubular heart forms, it begins to contract as

early as day 22 of development. The heart begins pumping blood about day 24, with the blood entering the sinus venosus and exiting the bulbus cordis.

Cardiac Looping

Cardiac looping is the first major step required for cardiac septation. This process essentially reverses the atrial and ventricular positions, moving the primitive atrium cranial and dorsal to the primitive ventricle. During looping, the bulbus cordis bends to the right, ventrally and inferiorly, while the primitive ventricle bends toward the left and somewhat dorsal to the bulbus cordis (**Part B**). Sometimes cardiac looping is reversed, thereby inverting the normal orientation of the mature heart. This condition is called dextrocardia.

Fate of Sinus Horns and Early Atrial Development

Before the atrium can be divided, all systemic venous blood must return to the right side of the primitive atrium. The opening of the sinus venosus shifts toward the right, mainly owing to cardiac looping, differential growth, and changes in hemodynamics (the left vitelline, umbilical, and common cardinal veins regress as venous anastomoses form elsewhere in the embryo) (**Part C**). Eventually, the left sinus horn regresses, with the remnant forming the coronary sinus. As the atrium expands, it incorporates the right sinus horn into its wall. The right common cardinal vein becomes the superior vena cava, and the right vitelline vein becomes the inferior vena cava. The right umbilical vein loses its connection to the sinus horn (see Chapter 37).

As the right atrium incorporates the sinus horn, a pair of tissue flaps develops on either side of the opening. The left fold is incorporated into the atrial septum, but the inferior right fold becomes the valve of the inferior vena cava and coronary sinus. The crista terminalis demarcates the junction between the original primitive atrium (trabecular part) and the smooth-walled sinus horn (sinus venarum). The crista terminalis carries fibers from the sinoatrial (SA) node to the atrioventricular (AV) node. The SA node differentiates from tissue in the right sinus horn near the common cardinal vein, and the AV node is thought to form from cells in the left sinus horn. The pulmonary veins sprout from the wall of the future left atrium, grow into the developing lung, and join blood vessels forming within the lung.

Clinical Aspects

Human left-right axis malformations are relatively rare. However, mirror-image reversal of all asymmetrical organs (heart, liver, stomach, intestines, etc.) is found and referred to as situs inversus (1/10,000 live births). Situs inversus is associated with immotile cilia syndrome, and affected individuals often have chronic respiratory infections, infertility, and ear infections. In contrast, if only some of the organs are reversed, the condition is referred to as situs ambiguus or heterotaxia. These individuals exhibit a broader range of anomalies, including heart defects that collectively can be fatal.

33 Heart II: Atrial Septation

A. Septation Process

1. Differential growth

Ridge · Muscular septum

2. Formation of cushion tissue (fibrous or membranous septa)

Endocardium
Myocardium
Cardiac jelly

New extracellular matrix

Myocardium

Superior endocardial cushion

Cushion cells

Cross section of heart between atrium and ventricle

Inferior endocardial cushion

3. Regions of cushion tissue formation

Aortic sac
Bulbus cordis

Bulbar cushion ridges
Primitive atrium
Sinus venosus
Atrioventricular canal
Inferior and superior cushion tissue
Primitive ventricle

B. Atrial Septation

33 days

Superior vena cava
Right atrium
Right endocardial cushion
Inferior vena cava
Inferior endocardial cushion of septum intermedium

Septum primum
Ostium primum
Left endocardial cushion
Ventricle

40 days

Superior vena cava
Right atrium
Ostium primum closing
Inferior vena cava
Right endocardial cushion
Inferior endocardial cushion

Septum secundum
Septum primum
Left atrium
Forming ostium secundum
Left endocardial cushion
Part of septum intermedium
Ventricle

43 days

Superior vena cava
Right atrium
Foramen ovale
Right endocardial cushion
Inferior endocardial cushion

Septum secundum
Septum primum
Left atrium
Ostium secundum
Left endocardial cushion
Ventricle
Muscular ventricular septum

C. Atrial Septal Defects and Valvular Defects

1. Normal septum formation

Septum secundum
Septum primum
Foramen ovale
Pulmonary veins
Ostium secundum

2. Excessive resorption of septum primum

Septum secundum
Pulmonary veins

3. Absence of septum secundum

Septum primum
Septum secundum

4. Patent ostium primum (low atrial septal defect)

Septum primum
Patent ostium primum

5. Absence of septum primum and septum secundum

6. Persistent atrioventricular canal (sagittal view)

Atrial septum
Atrial septal defect
Ventricular septal defect
Ventricular septum

7. Tricuspid atresia

Patent oval foramen
Pulmonary stenosis
Atresia of the cusps
Ventricular septal defect

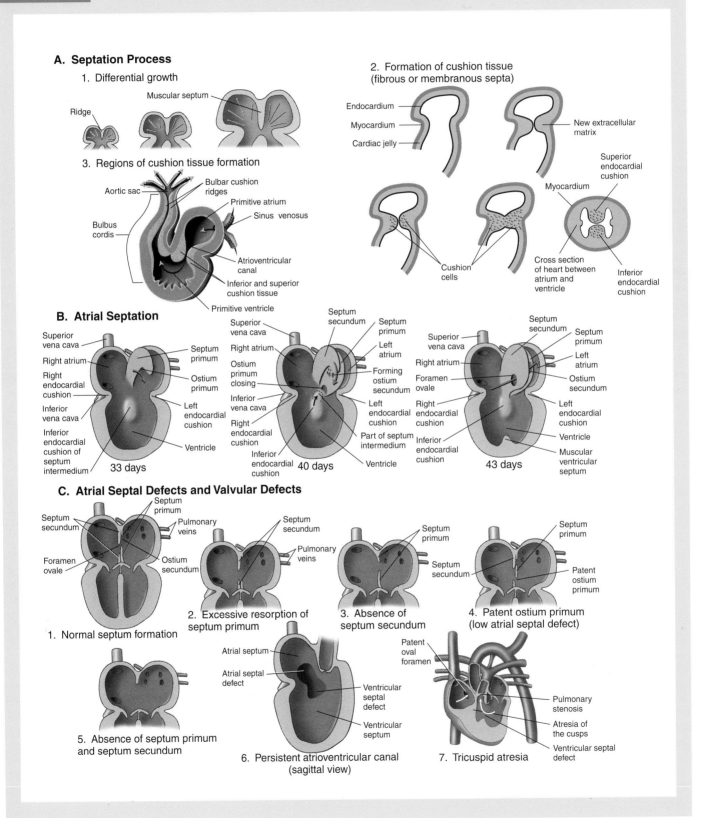

OVERVIEW

The septa of the heart consists of both muscular and fibrous portions. The muscular portion develops primarily through differential growth of the muscular walls during chamber expansion. The fibrous portion originates from cushion tissue. During atrial septation, 2 muscular septa form, septum primum and septum secundum. As ostium primum is closed by cushion tissue, ostium secundum develops within the upper part of septum primum but is overlapped by the growing septum secundum. Blood passes unilaterally from the right to the left atrium via the foramen ovale (os in septum secundum) but not the reverse, as septum primum together with septum secundum acts as a 1-way valve. Failure of septum primum and septum secundum formation, failure of cushion tissue formation, or development of an excessively large ostium secundum will result in atrial septal defects that, if not corrected, eventually lead to congestive heart failure.

Septation Process

Partitioning the heart into 4 chambers is accomplished through the formation of septa (walls) in the primitive atrium, ventricle, and bulbus cordis. Major events for cardiac septation occur between days 28 and 37 of gestation. Two basic processes are responsible for generating the septa (**Part A**). Differential growth, together with tissue remodeling, is primarily responsible for formation of the muscular portions of the interventricular and atrial septa. But this process never fully partitions the heart chambers. For that end, endocardial cushion tissue is required. In the atrioventricular and conotruncal regions, extracellular matrix is secreted between the endocardium and myocardium. Endocardial-derived mesenchymal cells then migrate and fill this space, forming new connective tissue. In the atrioventricular region, a superior and inferior expansion of cushion tissue fuses to form the septum intermedium, and this septum essentially separates the atrium and ventricle (**Part A**). This cushion tissue also contributes to the fibrous (membranous) portions of the interventricular and interatrial septa, the fibrous cardiac skeleton anchoring the heart valves, and the roots of the tricuspid and bicuspid valves. In the bulbus cordis region, cushion tissue forms as 2 ridges running along the entire length of the bulbus cordis. Eventually, these ridges fuse, separating the bulbus cordis into the aorta, pulmonary artery, and right ventricle (see Chapter 34). Mesenchymal cells in the conotruncal ridges are derived from 2 sources: the conotruncal endocardium and migrating neural crest cells from the aortic arches.

Atrial Septation

Separation of the atrium into 2 chambers requires that the atrial septum be leaky. If the left side is denied blood, the left ventricle becomes hypoplastic. Because the lungs are not fully developed or inflated, very little blood returns to the left atrium through this route. In addition, since oxygen-enriched placental blood enters the right atrium and ventricle, it is advantageous to skip the pulmonary system. Forming 2 septa solves the problem. During cardiac looping, the bulbus cordis induces the formation of septum primum (septum I). This growing sickle-shaped muscular septum extends from the atrial wall toward septum intermedium (**Part B**). Differential growth of the tissue alone is insufficient to fill the gap between septum primum and septum intermedium, leaving a hole called *ostium primum* (ostium I or foramen I). Upgrowth of cushion tissue from septum intermedium closes this hole as a second hole forms in the cranial part of septum primum called *ostium secundum* (ostium II or foramen II). Concurrently, another sickle-shaped and thicker septum forms, called *septum secundum* (septum II). Septum secundum overlaps ostium secundum but never completely separates the 2 atrial chambers. Rather, an opening called the *foramen ovale* remains within septum secundum, but this opening is overlapped by septum primum. During subsequent embryonic and fetal life, the thinner septum primum acts as a 1-way valve, allowing right atrial blood to enter the left atrium through the foramen ovale and ostium secundum. However, blood attempting to flow from left to right causes septum primum to press against septum secundum, sealing the foramen ovale.

After birth and with the first breath, the pulmonary circulation opens and blood flow increases through the lungs, increasing venous return to the left atrium. Because of deceased pulmonary resistance, both right atrial and ventricular pressures also drop. Consequently, pressure in the left cardiac chambers exceeds that in the right chambers, even during diastole. This drives septum primum against septum secundum, resulting in a functionally closed septum. Eventually the septa fuse (usually within 3 months after birth). Remnants of the foramen ovale (fossa ovalis) as well as ostium secundum can be found in the adult heart. In about 25% of the population, septum primum and secundum fail to close completely (probe patency), but this does not result in intracardiac shunting unless certain pathological conditions arise. Premature closure of the foramen ovale leads to right ventricular hypertrophy, left ventricular hypoplasia, and right-to-left shunting of blood through the ductus arteriosus. Depending on the degree of pathology, many of these newborns die unless they receive a heart transplant.

Atrial Septal Defects

The incidence of atrial septal defects is approximately 6–7/10,000, with a 2:1 prevalence in females versus males. At birth, most atrial septal defects result in an initial left-to-right shunt because of decreased pulmonary resistance once the lungs inflate. Over time, however, this leads to right ventricular hypertrophy and pulmonary congestion. As the right ventricle hypertrophies and the right intraventricular pressure increases, a right-to-left shunt eventually develops and signs of cyanosis may appear. Without intervention, the affected individual will die from congestive heart failure. High atrial septal defects can occur because of excessive resorption of septum primum creating an enlarged ostium secundum or because of inadequate development of septum secundum (**Part C**). Low septal defects can occur when cushion tissue from septum intermedium does not close ostium primum. Occasionally, a common atrium remains as neither septum primum nor septum secundum forms. In cases of persistent atrioventricular canal, septum intermedium does not form. Since this cushion tissue contributes to both atrial and ventricular septa, affected individuals have atrial and ventricular septal defects, valvular defects, and a common atrioventricular canal. Although this condition is rare, approximately 20% of patients with Down syndrome have this anomaly. Tricuspid atresia is an anomaly whereby the right atrioventricular orifice is obliterated. Fusion of the tricuspid valve primordia results in patency of the foramen ovale, ventricular septal defects, right ventricular hypoplasia, and left ventricular hypertrophy. This condition can be surgically corrected if the hypoplasia is not too severe.

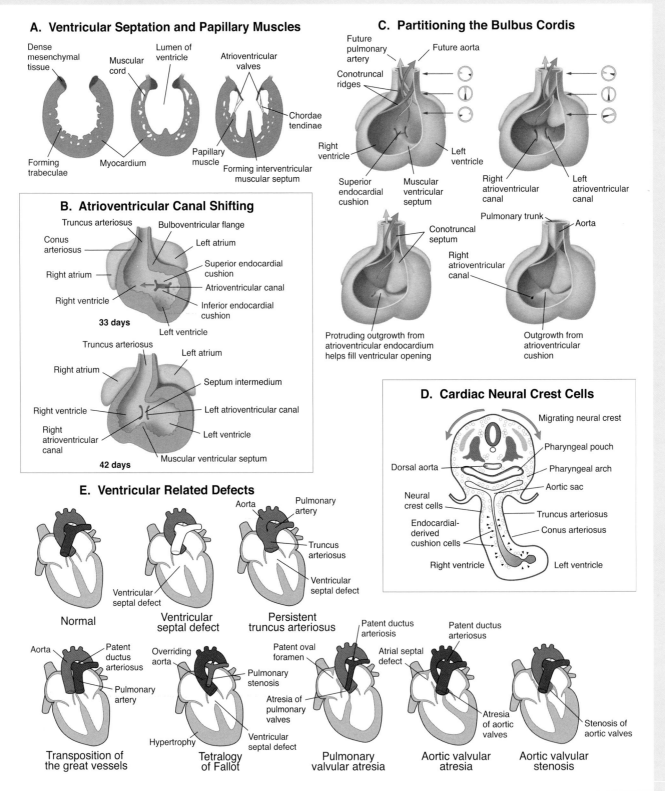

A. Ventricular Septation and Papillary Muscles

Dense mesenchymal tissue
Muscular cord
Lumen of ventricle
Atrioventricular valves
Chordae tendinae
Forming trabeculae
Myocardium
Papillary muscle
Forming interventricular muscular septum

B. Atrioventricular Canal Shifting

Truncus arteriosus
Bulboventricular flange
Conus arteriosus
Left atrium
Right atrium
Superior endocardial cushion
Atrioventricular canal
Right ventricle
Inferior endocardial cushion
Left ventricle

33 days

Truncus arteriosus
Left atrium
Right atrium
Septum intermedium
Right ventricle
Left atrioventricular canal
Right atrioventricular canal
Left ventricle
Muscular ventricular septum

42 days

C. Partitioning the Bulbus Cordis

Future pulmonary artery
Future aorta
Conotruncal ridges
Right ventricle
Left ventricle
Superior endocardial cushion
Muscular ventricular septum
Right atrioventricular canal
Left atrioventricular canal

Pulmonary trunk
Aorta
Conotruncal septum
Right atrioventricular canal

Protruding outgrowth from atrioventricular endocardium helps fill ventricular opening

Outgrowth from atrioventricular cushion

D. Cardiac Neural Crest Cells

Migrating neural crest
Pharyngeal pouch
Pharyngeal arch
Dorsal aorta
Aortic sac
Neural crest cells
Truncus arteriosus
Endocardial-derived cushion cells
Conus arteriosus
Right ventricle
Left ventricle

E. Ventricular Related Defects

Pulmonary artery
Aorta
Truncus arteriosus
Ventricular septal defect
Ventricular septal defect

Normal

Ventricular septal defect

Persistent truncus arteriosus

Aorta
Patent ductus arteriosus
Pulmonary artery

Overriding aorta
Pulmonary stenosis
Atresia of pulmonary valves
Hypertrophy
Ventricular septal defect

Patent ductus arteriosis
Patent oval foramen
Patent ductus arteriosus
Atrial septal defect
Atresia of aortic valves
Stenosis of aortic valves

Transposition of the great vessels

Tetralogy of Fallot

Pulmonary valvular atresia

Aortic valvular atresia

Aortic valvular stenosis

OVERVIEW

Dividing the primitive ventricle into right and left chambers requires formation of a muscular septum, formation and growth of septum intermedium, and division of the conotruncal segment. In order to connect the future aorta and pulmonary trunk with the appropriate chamber, the conotruncal septum must spiral before reaching the interventricular septum. Ventricular septal defects (VSDs) are the most common heart defect. Improper division of the conotruncal segment results in such defects as tetralogy of Fallot (unequal conotruncal division), transposition of the great vessels (failure of the conotruncal septum to spiral), persistent truncus arteriosus (absence of the conotruncal septum), and semilunar valvular defects (improper development of cushion tissue at the conal-truncal interface). Because neural crest cells are an important source of conotruncal cushion cells, many congenital heart defects are now considered neurocristopathies.

Ventricular Septation

As the primitive left and right ventricles expand, their luminal surfaces develop muscular infoldings called *trabeculae,* and some are remodeled to form the papillary muscles (**Part A**). As the atrioventricular valves form, the valve leaflets remain attached to some of these papillary muscles via cords that eventually become the chordae tendineae. In order to deliver blood into both the future right and left ventricles, the atrioventricular canal shifts toward the right so that the forming septum intermedium becomes aligned with the forming interventricular septum (**Part B**). As the primitive ventricle expands, the muscular portion forms by differential growth. And, like the atrium, closure of the interventricular foramen requires cushion tissue originating from septum intermedium and from the conotruncal septum.

Partitioning of the Bulbus Cordis

The truncus arteriosus is divided into the aorta and pulmonary artery, while the conus segment connects the future ventricles to these arteries. The right ventricle connects to the right and left aortic arch 6 (pulmonary circulation), and the left ventricle connects to aortic arches 3 and 4 (systemic circulation). To accomplish this, 2 opposing ridges of cushion tissue form along the entire length of the conotruncal segment and fuse, forming the conotruncal septum and thereby dividing the outflow tract into 2 vessels (**Part C**). However, rather than running straight down from the aortic sac toward the ventricle, these ridges spiral 180 degrees and end up perfectly aligned with the interventricular septum and septum intermedium, connecting the right ventricle with the future pulmonary trunk and the left ventricle with the future aorta. The conotruncal septum also contributes to the closure of the interventricular foramen. Eventually, the proximal roots of the aorta and pulmonary trunk are incorporated into the 2 expanding ventricles. Semilunar valves form at the truncal-conal junction by remodeling and sculpting of the conotruncal septum. Whereas cushion cells of septum intermedium are derived from endocardium, cushion cells in the bulbus cordis are derived from 2 sources, conotruncal endocardium and neural crest cells (**Part D**). Therefore, factors that perturb the morphogenesis of neural crest cells significantly increase the risk of cardiac defects.

VSDs and Great Vessel Anomalies

The incidence of VSDs is 12–15/10,000, making them the most common congenital heart defect in live births (**Part E**). Complete closure requires the septum intermedium, proper development of the conotruncal septum, and the interventricular muscular septum. Approximately 95% of VSDs involve improper development of the nonmuscular portion. Infants born with VSDs often exhibit initial left-to-right shunting of blood and are acyanotic. However, as right ventricular hypertrophy and pulmonary congestion progress, right-to-left shunting eventually ensues and cyanosis appears. Without surgical intervention these individuals eventually die from congestive heart failure. Progression of the disease varies, depending on the size of the VSD and whether it is accompanied by other defects.

Several cardiac anomalies arise due to improper septation of the bulbus cordis (**Part E**). When the conotruncal ridges fail to form or fuse, the result is persistent truncus arteriosus (1/10,000 births). Here, the pulmonary artery and aorta arise downstream from an undivided truncus arteriosus, and a VSD develops because the conotruncal component of the interventricular septum is absent. A left-to-right shunt ensues at birth but eventually cyanosis develops as pulmonary congestion and right ventricular hypertrophy progress. Occasionally, the conotruncal ridges form and fuse but fail to spiral. Consequently, the pulmonary artery and aorta are connected to the wrong ventricles, forming a condition known as *transposition of the great vessels* (incidence of 5/10,000). These newborns survive only because of vascular shunts (VSD, atrial septal defects, or a patent ductus arteriosus), for these shunts provide the only means of channeling blood to the pulmonary circulation. Even with shunts, the life expectancy is 6 months to 3 years without surgery. If the conotruncal ridges do not equally divide the lumen of the outflow tract, then pulmonary stenosis, an overriding aorta, and a VSD result. Newborns with this condition have tetralogy of Fallot (9–10/10,000). Pulmonary stenosis and the VSD lead to fetal right ventricular hypertrophy that usually has progressed to the point that right-to-left shunts and cyanosis can be present at birth. Tetralogy of Fallot is the most common congenital heart defect resulting in cyanosis at birth.

Valvular Defects

Valvular defects also result from improper remodeling of the bulbus cordis (3–4/10,000) (**Part E**). Atresia of the pulmonary semilunar valves leads to right ventricular hypoplasia as blood will not flow into this chamber. A patent foramen ovale develops because it is the only outlet for the systemic venous blood to get to the systemic arterial side. The ductus arteriosus is also patent as it is the only route for blood to get to the lungs. With aortic valvular atresia, the left ventricle is severely hypoplastic. Because the right ventricle carries the entire workload during fetal life, it is hypertrophied. A wide ductus arteriosus usually develops, as it is the only means for oxygen-enriched blood from the placenta to get into the left systemic side. After birth, oxygen-enriched blood must enter the right atrium by way of an atrial septal defect and then into the systemic circulation by passing through a patent ductus arteriosus. This condition is usually not compatible with life without a heart transplantation. Occasionally, stenosis of the aortic semilunar valves occurs, leading to hypertrophy of the left ventricle and eventual cardiac failure if not corrected.

The fibrous portions of the cushion-derived tissue surrounding the roots of the valves electrically isolate the atria from the ventricles. The myocardium in this region disappears by an unknown mechanism. Wolff-Parkinson-White syndrome (1–2/1,000 live births) is a condition whereby residual myocardium persists in this area, leading to dysrhythmias.

Vascular Development I: Arteries

A. Primitive Arteries & Veins

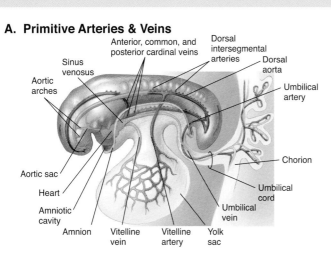

B. Intersegmental & Aortic Arch Arteries

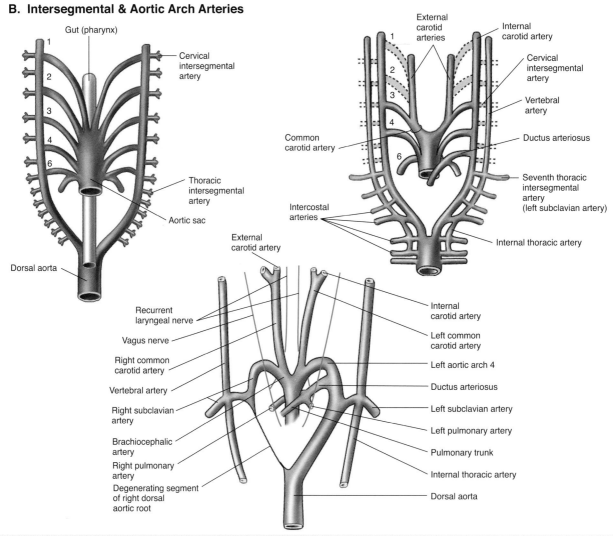

OVERVIEW

The adult great arteries are produced by modifying a system of primitive vessels consisting of aortic arches, paired dorsal aortae, and intersegmental arteries. Three major types of modifications occur: (1) hypertrophy of some vessels, (2) addition of new vessels, and (3) loss of some vessel segments. Five pairs of primitive vessels form within the pharyngeal arches that connect the paired cranial dorsal aortae to the aortic sac found at the downstream end of the primitive heart. Aortic arches 3 and 4 are major contributors to the adult aortic arch and large systemic arteries, while aortic arch 6 connects the pulmonary artery to the lungs. Aortic arches 1 and 2 regress. At the caudal end of the fused dorsal aortae, vitelline and umbilical arteries develop that supply the gastrointestinal tract and send blood to the placenta.

The Primitive Arterial System

As the primitive heart moves into the thoracic region, it pulls the cranial end of each developing dorsal aorta along with it, thereby forming the first pair of aortic arches. Five additional pairs of aortic arches eventually connect the cardiac aortic sac to the dorsal aortae (**Part A**), and these form within the pharyngeal arches of the head and neck (see Chapter 22). The adult pattern of great arteries is produced by basic alterations of this primitive system through 3 major processes: (1) hypertrophy of some vessels, (2) addition of new vessels, and (3) a loss of some vessel segments. Development of these arteries in a normal pattern requires interactions with neural crest–derived mesenchyme in the pharyngeal arches.

Dorsal Intersegmental Arteries

New vessels emerge from the right and left dorsal aortae that extend laterally between the somites (**Part B**). These intersegmental arteries develop anastomoses along the cranial-caudal axis. Once established, the first 6 cervical intersegmental arteries regress, and the remaining anastomoses form the vertebral arteries. Thoracic intersegmental arteries and additional anastomoses lead to formation of the intercostal arteries, the internal thoracic, superior and inferior epigastric, deep cervical, and superior intercostal arteries. The lumbar and sacral intersegmental arteries form the lumbar and lateral sacral arteries.

Fate of Aortic Arches (Part B)

Aortic arches 1 and 2: These 2 vessels regress, but some cells contribute to the maxillary and stapedial arteries.

Aortic arch 3: This aortic arch forms the common carotid artery and the proximal portion of the internal carotid artery. The remainder of the internal carotid develops from the cranial dorsal aorta. The external carotid forms from remnants of the cranial aortic sac after aortic arches 1 and 2 regress. The external carotid remains connected to aortic arch 3.

Left aortic arch 4: Left aortic arch 4 forms a portion of the adult aortic arch. The adult aortic arch develops from the aortic sac, left aortic arch 4, left dorsal aorta proximal to the seventh intersegmental artery, and left dorsal aorta distal to the seventh intersegmental artery. The left seventh intersegmental artery forms the left subclavian artery. The conotruncal septum ensures that the adult aortic arch connects to the left ventricle.

Right aortic arch 4: The right seventh dorsal intersegmental artery forms the distal portion of the right subclavian artery, and the right aortic arch 4 and intervening dorsal aorta make up the proximal portion. The aortic sac remodels to eventually form a common trunk for right aortic arches 3 and 4 that is called the *brachiocephalic artery*.

Aortic arch 5: This arch regresses.

Aortic arch 6: The right and left aortic arch 6 form new vascular branches that enter the lung and connect to the developing intrapulmonary vasculature. Once connected, the distal portion of the right aortic arch 6 (adjacent to the dorsal aorta) regresses, but the left one is retained as the *ductus arteriosus*. Initially, the heart begins developing within the cervical region but ends up within the thorax. As the heart descends, the roots of the common carotid and subclavian arteries elongate and descend with it. The intrinsic musculature of the larynx is derived from mesenchyme of the sixth pharyngeal arch, and its vagal innervation is established early. Therefore, as the heart descends, the vagal branches supplying the larynx are also dragged down with the heart. Since the distal segment of the right aortic arch 6 arch is lost, the right recurrent nerve becomes hooked under the right subclavian artery (right aortic arch 4). On the left, the recurrent laryngeal nerve becomes hooked under ductus arteriosus (left aortic arch 6), which eventually regresses to form the *ligamentum arteriosum*.

Primitive dorsal aorta: The paired primitive dorsal aortae fuse to make a single vessel in the lower thorax and abdomen. The segments of the dorsal aortae between aortic arches 3 and 4 are eventually obliterated as is the distal right dorsal aortic segment between the right seventh intersegmental artery and thoracic aorta.

Vitelline and Umbilical Arteries

The vitelline arteries supplying the yolk sac connect to the dorsal aorta and form the celiac, superior mesenteric, and inferior mesenteric arteries. The umbilical arteries form as branches from the dorsal aortae coursing to the placenta but eventually become connected to the fifth lumbar intersegmental arteries (future iliac artery). At birth, the distal ends of the umbilical arteries regress and become the medial umbilical ligaments, while the proximal ends become the superior vesicular arteries supplying the bladder.

Vascular Development II: Congenital Anomalies of the Great Arteries

A. Patent Ductus Arteriosus

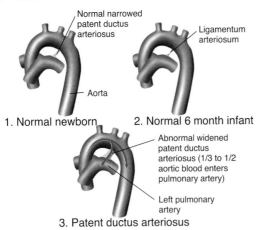

Normal narrowed patent ductus arteriosus

Ligamentum arteriosum

Aorta

1. Normal newborn

2. Normal 6 month infant

Abnormal widened patent ductus arteriosus (1/3 to 1/2 aortic blood enters pulmonary artery)

Left pulmonary artery

3. Patent ductus arteriosus

B. Coarctation of the Aorta

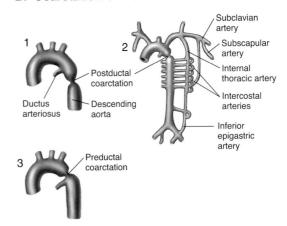

1

2

Postductal coarctation

Ductus arteriosus

Descending aorta

Subclavian artery

Subscapular artery

Internal thoracic artery

Intercostal arteries

Inferior epigastric artery

3

Preductal coarctation

C. Other Anomalies of the Great Vessels

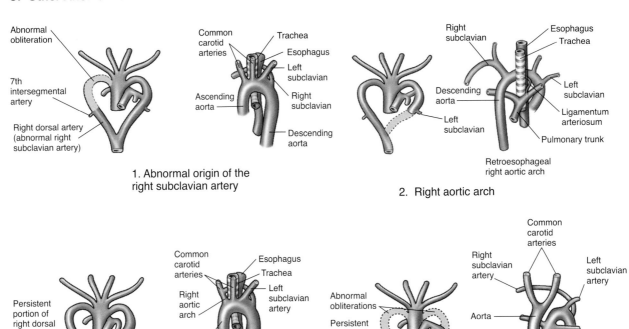

Abnormal obliteration

7th intersegmental artery

Right dorsal artery (abnormal right subclavian artery)

1. Abnormal origin of the right subclavian artery

Common carotid arteries

Trachea

Esophagus

Left subclavian

Ascending aorta

Right subclavian

Descending aorta

Right subclavian

Descending aorta

Left subclavian

Esophagus

Trachea

Left subclavian

Ligamentum arteriosum

Pulmonary trunk

Retroesophageal right aortic arch

2. Right aortic arch

Persistent portion of right dorsal aorta

Common carotid arteries

Esophagus

Trachea

Left subclavian artery

Right aortic arch

Descending aorta

Ascending aorta

3. Double aortic arch

Abnormal obliterations

Persistent portion of right dorsal aorta

Common carotid arteries

Right subclavian artery

Left subclavian artery

Aorta

Pulmonary artery

4. Interrupted aortic arch

OVERVIEW

Abnormal retention and loss of various segments of the aortic arches result in blood vessel anomalies that may or may not be symptomatic. Abnormal narrowing of the aorta (coarctation) proximal (upstream) to the ductus arteriosus can lead to differential cyanosis in postnatal life, whereas coarctation distal to the ductus arteriosus is usually asymptomatic. A patent ductus arteriosus (failure to close the shunt between the pulmonary artery and aorta) leads to right ventricular hypertension if not corrected. Other anomalies of the arteries can be life-threatening or have implications in surgery and diagnosis.

Congenital Anomalies of the Great Arteries

The postnatal and adult vasculature develops from the remodeling of a primitive vasculature. This remodeling includes the loss, retention, or addition of new vascular elements. Therefore, development of the arterial system is prone to variation. Many of these variations are asymptomatic. However, anomalies that are clinically relevant do occur, some of which can be life-threatening.

Patent Ductus Arteriosus

Shortly after birth, the ductus arteriosus closes through contraction of its muscular wall (**Part A**). If it remains open (8/10,000 births), one-third to one-half of the aortic blood enters the pulmonary artery because the systemic pressure exceeds the pulmonary pressure. The re-entry into the lungs increases venous return to the left atrium and ventricle, causing left ventricular hypertrophy, increased pulmonary resistance, and eventual right ventricular hypertension.

Coarctation of the Aorta

The aortic lumen below the origin of the left subclavian artery can narrow owing to abnormal thickening of the aortic wall, and the narrowing may occur proximal or distal to the ductus arteriosus (3/10,000 births) (**Part B**). Postductal coarctation may be asymptomatic as collateral circulation is established during embryonic and fetal life. However, with preductal coarctation the collateral circulation is not well developed as oxygen- and nutrient-enriched blood from the placenta reaches the lower portion of the body via the ductus arteriosus. After birth, the ductus arteriosus remains patent, supplying only venous blood from the right ventricle to the lower body. This can lead to differential cyanosis, whereby the upper part of the body is normal in color, while the lower part is cyanotic. If preductal coarctation is pronounced, affected children often die without surgery.

Anomalous Right Subclavian Artery

The right subclavian artery usually forms from the right aortic arch 4, proximal right dorsal aorta, and seventh intersegmental artery, while the distal segment of the right dorsal aorta is lost. In some individuals, the proximal segment is lost and the distal right dorsal aorta is retained, resulting in an anomalous origin of the right subclavian artery (**Part C**). These patients can exhibit difficulties in swallowing (dysphagia) and breathing (dysapnea) as the right subclavian artery crosses behind the esophagus and trachea to reach the aorta on the left.

Right Aortic Arch

Occasionally, the left aortic arch 4 and the left dorsal aorta are obliterated and replaced by corresponding vessels on the right (**Part C**). If the ductus arteriosus forms between the right aortic arch 6 (future right pulmonary artery) and the right dorsal aorta, no vascular ring forms. This condition is usually asymptomatic. However, if the ductus arteriosus forms on the left side, it will form a vascular ring. These patients may complain of dysphagia because the ligamentum arteriosum passes behind the esophagaus toward the right.

Double Aortic Arch

If the right distal dorsal aorta does not regress, it forms a vascular ring surrounding the trachea and esophagus (**Part C**). This may lead to esophageal dysfunction and difficulty in breathing.

Interrupted Aortic Arch

A very serious condition results when the right and left aortic arch 4 disappear (**Part C**). The ductus arteriosus remains patent, and the descending aorta and subclavian arteries are supplied with blood of low oxygen content. The aortic trunk only supplies the 2 common carotid arteries. This also leads to differential cyanosis.

37 Vascular Development III: Veins

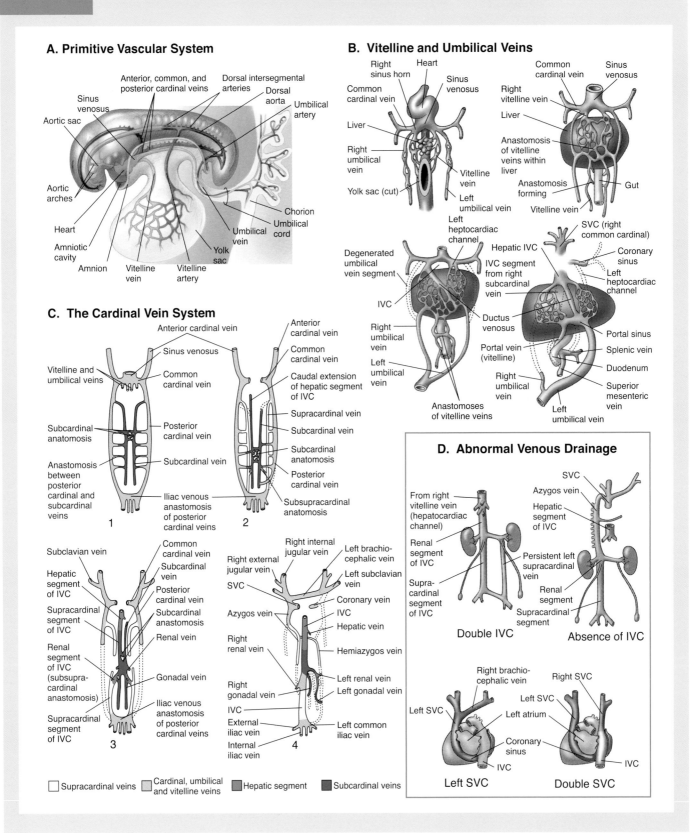

A. Primitive Vascular System

Anterior, common, and posterior cardinal veins
Dorsal intersegmental arteries
Sinus venosus
Dorsal aorta
Aortic sac
Umbilical artery
Aortic arches
Heart
Amniotic cavity
Amnion
Vitelline vein
Vitelline artery
Yolk sac
Umbilical vein
Umbilical cord
Chorion

B. Vitelline and Umbilical Veins

Right sinus horn
Heart
Common cardinal vein
Sinus venosus
Liver
Right umbilical vein
Vitelline vein
Yolk sac (cut)
Left umbilical vein

Common cardinal vein
Sinus venosus
Right vitelline vein
Liver
Anastomosis of vitelline veins within liver
Anastomosis forming
Gut
Vitelline vein

Left heptocardiac channel
Degenerated umbilical vein segment
IVC
Right umbilical vein
Left umbilical vein
Ductus venosus
Portal vein (vitelline)
Right umbilical vein
Anastomoses of vitelline veins
Left umbilical vein

Hepatic IVC
IVC segment from right subcardinal vein
SVC (right common cardinal)
Coronary sinus
Left heptocardiac channel
Portal sinus
Splenic vein
Duodenum
Superior mesenteric vein

C. The Cardinal Vein System

Anterior cardinal vein
Sinus venosus
Vitelline and umbilical veins
Common cardinal vein
Subcardinal anatomosis
Posterior cardinal vein
Anastomosis between posterior cardinal and subcardinal veins
Subcardinal vein
Iliac venous anastomosis of posterior cardinal veins
1

Anterior cardinal vein
Common cardinal vein
Caudal extension of hepatic segment of IVC
Supracardinal vein
Subcardinal vein
Subcardinal anatomosis
Posterior cardinal vein
Subsupracardinal anatomosis
2

Subclavian vein
Common cardinal vein
Subcardinal vein
Hepatic segment of IVC
Posterior cardinal vein
Supracardinal segment of IVC
Subcardinal anastomosis
Renal vein
Renal segment of IVC (subsupracardinal anastomosis)
Gonadal vein
Iliac venous anastomosis of posterior cardinal veins
Supracardinal segment of IVC
3

Right internal jugular vein
Right external jugular vein
Left brachiocephalic vein
SVC
Left subclavian vein
Coronary vein
Azygos vein
IVC
Hepatic vein
Right renal vein
Hemiazygos vein
Left renal vein
Right gonadal vein
Left gonadal vein
IVC
External iliac vein
Internal iliac vein
Left common iliac vein
4

D. Abnormal Venous Drainage

From right vitelline vein (hepatocardiac channel)
Renal segment of IVC
Supracardinal segment of IVC
Double IVC

SVC
Azygos vein
Hepatic segment of IVC
Persistent left supracardinal vein
Renal segment
Supracardinal segment
Absence of IVC

Right brachiocephalic vein
Left SVC
Left SVC
Left atrium
Coronary sinus
IVC

Right SVC
Left SVC
Double SVC
Left atrium
IVC

☐ Supracardinal veins ☐ Cardinal, umbilical and vitelline veins ■ Hepatic segment ■ Subcardinal veins

OVERVIEW

The major veins in the body are derived from 3 basic sets of primitive vessels, the vitelline veins, umbilical veins, and cardinal veins. The vitelline veins carry blood back from the developing GI tract and contribute to the portal system and a segment of the inferior vena cava. The umbilical veins carry blood from the placenta through the liver and eventually regress. The common cardinal system carries blood from the remainder of the body and has 2 main trunks, the anterior and posterior cardinal veins. Originally, the embryo starts with separate right and left sets of veins. However, venous return to the heart is shifted to the right side through the formation of anastomoses and a corresponding loss of longitudinal venous segments on the left side. Formation of the final adult venous system generally encompasses the same basic mechanisms as those used in the formation of the arterial system; however, it is prone to greater variation, many of which are asymptomatic.

Early Venous System

Early in development, 3 sets of primitive veins form, the right and left vitelline veins, umbilical veins, and common cardinal veins (**Part A**). These primitive vessels collect and deliver venous blood back to the right and left sinus horns of the sinus venosus, which empty into the primitive atrium. As discussed in Chapter 32, the opening of the sinus venosus shifts toward the right side of the primitive atrium, while the left sinus horn begins regressing as anastomoses develop between the right and left venous systems. All venous return is then shunted toward the right side. The vitelline veins carry blood from the yolk sac, the umbilical veins carry oxygen-rich blood from the placenta, the cardinal system (anterior and posterior) drains the main body of the embryo, and all of them deliver venous blood to the sinus horns.

Vitelline Veins

The vitelline veins develop within the septum transversum and become surrounded by the liver primordia (**Part B**). As the liver develops, the vitelline veins form a vascular plexus (hepatic sinusoids) within the liver primordia. As the left sinus horn regresses, blood flow from the left vitelline is channeled toward the right side within the liver. Meanwhile, the proximal-most segment of the right vitelline vein enlarges and forms the right hepatocardiac channel. This segment eventually forms the terminal part of the inferior vena cava. The proximal part of the left vitelline vein then disappears. The more distal (caudal) segments of the vitelline veins regress, except for parts that contribute to the portal, superior and inferior mesenteric, and splenic veins.

Umbilical Veins

Meanwhile, the umbilical veins, passing on either side of the developing liver, establish a connection with the hepatic sinusoids (**Part B**). The proximal segments between the new connections and the sinus horns regress, as does the distal right umbilical vein. With increased placental circulation, a more direct communication is formed between the incoming left umbilical vein and the right hepatocardiac channel. This channel is called the *ductus venosus*. Since the maternal liver has already processed many of the nutrients, most of the placental blood bypasses the sinusoidal plexus of the liver. After birth, the left umbilical vein and ductus venosus regress, forming the *ligamentum teres hepatis* and *ligamentum venosum*, respectively.

Cardinal System

The anterior and posterior cardinal veins are the early drainage system for the entire body, excluding the developing portal system. Both cardinal veins join together before entering the sinus horn and forming the common cardinal vein (**Part C**). Anastomoses develop between the left and right anterior and posterior cardinal veins, so that eventually all venous blood drains primarily into the right cardinal system.

Anterior Cardinal System

The anterior cardinal veins drain the head, neck, upper limbs, and upper thorax. The superior vena cava develops from the union of the proximal right anterior cardinal vein and the right common cardinal vein (**Part C**). An anastomosis develops between the right and left anterior cardinal veins, forming the left brachiocephalic vein. A short right brachiocephalic vein forms from the junction of the proximal right subclavian vein and internal jugular, which then joins the left brachiocephalic vein at the superior vena cava. Meanwhile, on the left, the connection between the left anterior cardinal and the left common cardinal vein disappears, and the left sinus horn regresses, forming the coronary sinus and a remnant vein on the heart surface called the *oblique vein*.

Posterior Cardinal System

Posterior cardinal veins are the primitive veins draining the lower thoracic wall, abdomen, pelvis, and lower limbs (**Part C**). Two additional vein systems develop parallel to the posterior cardinals and anastomose with the posterior cardinal veins. The subcardinal veins are primarily associated with the kidney and gonads and contribute to a segment of the inferior vena cava. The supracardinal veins primarily drain the posterior body wall and contribute to the formation of the lower inferior vena cava and to the azygos system.

Inferior Vena Cava

The inferior vena cava (**Part C**) is derived from (1) the right hepatocardiac channel; (2) the right subcardinal vein between the liver and the kidney; (3) the renal segment (from the right subcardinal-supracardinal anastomosis); and (4) the lower segment of the right supracardinal vein.

Abnormal Venous Drainage (Part D)

Double inferior vena cava: The left supracardinal vein retains its connection with the left subcardinal vein. The left common iliac vein may or may not be present.

Absence of inferior vena cava: The right subcardinal vein fails to connect with the right hepatocardiac segment, and consequently venous blood is alternatively shunted into the right supracardinal vein. Hence, blood from the caudal part of the body reaches the heart by way of the azygos vein, while the hepatic vein empties directly into the right atrium rather than the inferior vena cava.

Left superior vena cava: The left anterior and common cardinal veins persist, with a concomitant loss of the right common and proximal right anterior cardinal veins. Venous blood from the right side is channeled toward the left by way of a long right brachiocephalic vein. Blood in the left superior vena cava drains into the right atrium by way of the coronary sinus. Left superior vena cava is usually found in patients with situs inversus.

Double superior vena cava: The left brachiocephalic vein does not form; thus, the entire left anterior and common cardinal veins persist. The persistent left anterior and common cardinal veins form a left superior vena cava that drains into the right atrium by way of the coronary sinus.

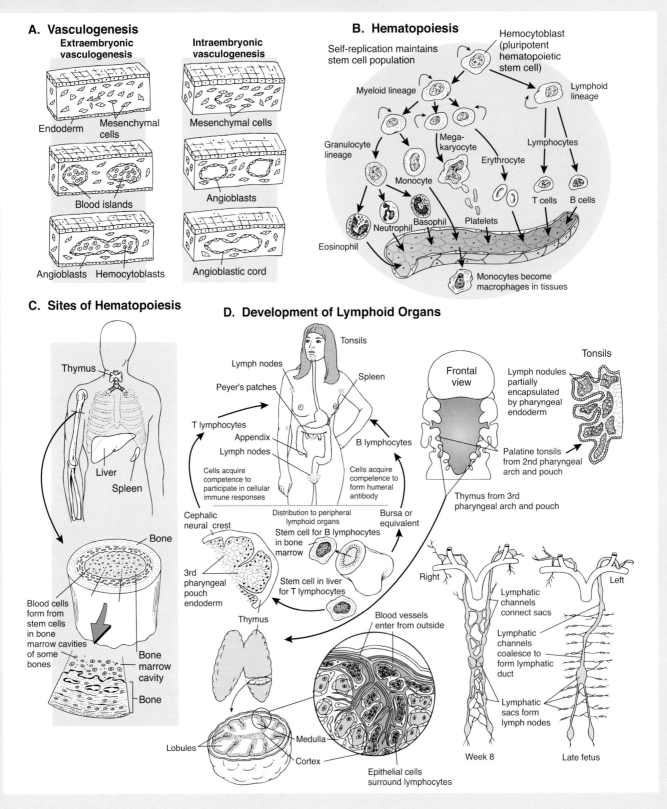

A. Vasculogenesis

Extraembryonic vasculogenesis

Endoderm — Mesenchymal cells

Blood islands

Angioblasts   Hemocytoblasts

Intraembryonic vasculogenesis

Mesenchymal cells

Angioblasts

Angioblastic cord

B. Hematopoiesis

Hemocytoblast (pluripotent hematopoietic stem cell)

Self-replication maintains stem cell population

Myeloid lineage

Lymphoid lineage

Granulocyte lineage

Mega-karyocyte

Lymphocytes

Erythrocyte

Monocyte

T cells   B cells

Eosinophil

Neutrophil   Basophil   Platelets

Monocytes become macrophages in tissues

C. Sites of Hematopoiesis

Thymus

Liver

Spleen

Bone

Blood cells form from stem cells in bone marrow cavities of some bones

Bone marrow cavity

Bone

D. Development of Lymphoid Organs

Tonsils

Lymph nodes

Peyer's patches

Spleen

T lymphocytes

Appendix

Lymph nodes

B lymphocytes

Cells acquire competence to participate in cellular immune responses

Cells acquire competence to form humeral antibody

Distribution to peripheral lymphoid organs

Cephalic neural crest

Bursa or equivalent

Stem cell for B lymphocytes in bone marrow

3rd pharyngeal pouch endoderm

Stem cell in liver for T lymphocytes

Thymus

Lobules

Medulla

Cortex

Blood vessels enter from outside

Epithelial cells surround lymphocytes

Frontal view

Thymus from 3rd pharyngeal arch and pouch

Tonsils

Lymph nodules partially encapsulated by pharyngeal endoderm

Palatine tonsils from 2nd pharyngeal arch and pouch

Right

Left

Lymphatic channels connect sacs

Lymphatic channels coalesce to form lymphatic duct

Lymphatic sacs form lymph nodes

Week 8

Late fetus

OVERVIEW

Vasculogenesis is the process of forming blood vessels directly from mesoderm. It begins in the extraembryonic mesoderm of the yolk sac, where it is coupled with hematopoiesis. In contrast, intraembryonic vasculogenesis is not coupled with hematopoiesis. The earliest hemopoietic stem cells are hemocytoblasts, and they produce lymphoid and myeloid stem cells. The yolk sac is the earliest site of hematopoiesis, but eventually it shifts to the liver and spleen and then to the bone marrow. Hematopoietic stem cells populate and contribute to the development of various lymphoid tissues, including the lymph nodes, tonsils, spleen, and thymus.

Early Vasculogenesis

The formation of blood vessels directly from mesoderm is called *vasculogenesis*. The earliest vasculogenesis is coupled with hematopoiesis (blood cell formation). Beginning on day 17, cells within the yolk sac splanchnic mesoderm form hemangioblasts (**Part A**). Hemangioblasts then differentiate into hemocytoblasts (blood stem cells) and angioblasts. Angioblasts differentiate into endothelial cells and, together with the hemocytoblasts, form blood islands. Blood islands coalesce, lengthen, and interconnect to form the first blood vessels. By the end of the third week, a vascularized yolk sac wall, connecting stalk, and chorionic villi are formed. Therefore, these tissue sites are the first hematopoietic organs.

Intraembryonic vasculogenesis is not coupled with hematopoiesis (**Part A**). Aggregates of angioblasts organize into small vesicle-like structures that coalesce to form long hollow cords of blood vessels. The angioplastic plexus grows and spreads by (1) continued formation and fusion of angioblast aggregates; (2) angiogenesis, the budding and sprouting of new vessels from existing ones; and (3) recruitment of mesodermal cells into the vessel walls.

Hematopoiesis

Stem cells generate a self-renewing source of parental cells and a daughter cell subpopulation that go on to the next phase of differentiation. For blood cells, the earliest stem cells are called *hemocytoblasts* (or pluripotent hematopoietic stem cells). Hemocytoblasts undergo massive cell proliferation and produce all blood cell types (**Part B**). Hemocytoblast daughter cells produce 2 basic cell lineages, lymphoid stem cells (which eventually produce B and T lymphocytes) and myeloid stem cells (which eventually produce erythrocytes, granulocytes, monocytes, and megakaryocytes). Formation of specific cell types is regulated at each step by specific colony-stimulating factors.

Organ Sites for Hematopoieses

Blood islands in the yolk sac and extraembryonic mesoderm contain hemocytoblasts and produce all cell types found in the embryonic blood. However, by the fifth to sixth week, the liver begins functioning as a hematopoietic organ (**Part C**). The spleen also becomes a site of hematopoiesis (see below). Hematopoiesis continues in the liver until the neonatal period, by which time it completely shifts to the bone marrow. Cortisol synthesized by the fetal adrenal cortex is thought to mediate this shift.

Spleen

The spleen develops within the splanchnic mesoderm sandwiched between layers of the dorsal mesentery that attach the stomach to the body wall (dorsal mesogastrium). The mesoderm produces the stromal network and capsule of the spleen and is subsequently invaded by developing blood vessels. Hemocytoblasts populate the splenic primordia and take up residence. Splenic hematopoiesis is mostly limited to producing RBCs and usually ceases late in the fetal period.

Tonsils

The tonsils form within the pharyngeal wall. Tonsilar connective tissue is derived from mesoderm and neural crest cells. In the case of palatine tonsils, the mesenchyme is derived from pharyngeal arch 2 and covered by pharyngeal pouch 2 endoderm (see Chapter 24 and **Part D**). Lymphocytes invade the connective tissue framework during the second month. The other tonsils are derived through a similar process.

Thymus

The thymus is the site where thymic precursor cells (thymocytes) become committed and transformed into immunocompetent T cells. These T cells are then exported to other lymphoid organs. The thymus gland is segregated into lobules, each consisting of a cortex and medulla made of epithelial stromal cells surrounded by lymphocytes (**Part D**). Thymic development begins when endodermal cells from the third and possibly fourth pair of pharyngeal pouches separate and migrate toward the sternum (see Chapter 24). The endodermal cells interact with neural crest cells and differentiate into the epithelial stromal cells, while neural crest cells form the capsule and septa of the thymus. Thymocyte precursors from the liver enter the thymic primordia, and the stromal cells stimulate thymocyte proliferation. Exposure to various thymic hormones transforms the thymocyte precursors into immunocompetent T cells that then populate other organs. B cells undergo a similar conditioning, but it is thought to occur within the bone marrow.

Lymphatic Vessels

The formation of lymphatic vessels is thought to be similar to that of blood vessels. Primary lymph vessel sacs appear during the sixth week, including 2 jugular lymph sacs (near the future internal jugular vein), retroperitoneal sacs (in the posterior body wall), cisterna chyli (dorsal to the aorta), and posterior lymph sacs (along the femoral and sciatic veins). These sacs become interconnected by developing lymphatic vessels and connect to the cisterna chyli (**Part D**). Eventually, these vessels are remodeled into a single lymphatic vessel (the thoracic duct) that empties into the left subclavian vein.

Clinical Aspects

Capillary hemangiomas, particularly of the skin (birthmarks), result from abnormal vasculogenesis and angiogenesis of the capillaries. Hemangiomas may be physically harmless or grow to form vascular tangles with clinical consequences (e.g., in the brain, where tangles can restrict blood flow). Congenital lymphedema is a condition characterized by diffuse swelling due to hypoplasia of the lymphatic vessels. Cystic hygroma is a condition present at birth whereby the lymphatic vessels are dilated, producing a swollen appearance at the root of the neck. Immunodeficiency accompanies DiGeorge syndrome (see Chapter 24). Umbilical cord blood contains primitive hematopoietic stem cells. These cells have been used in the treatment of diseases normally requiring bone marrow transplantation.

39 The Integument

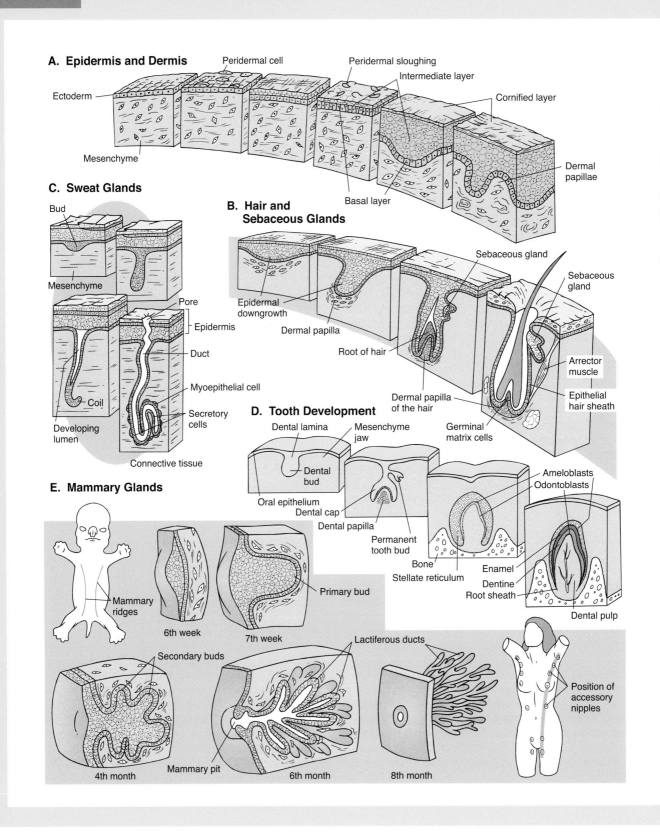

A. Epidermis and Dermis

Ectoderm
Peridermal cell
Peridermal sloughing
Intermediate layer
Cornified layer
Mesenchyme
Dermal papillae
Basal layer

C. Sweat Glands

Bud
Mesenchyme
Pore
Epidermis
Duct
Myoepithelial cell
Coil
Secretory cells
Developing lumen
Connective tissue

B. Hair and Sebaceous Glands

Epidermal downgrowth
Dermal papilla
Root of hair
Dermal papilla of the hair
Germinal matrix cells
Sebaceous gland
Sebaceous gland
Arrector muscle
Epithelial hair sheath

D. Tooth Development

Dental lamina
Mesenchyme jaw
Dental bud
Oral epithelium
Dental cap
Dental papilla
Permanent tooth bud
Bone
Stellate reticulum
Ameloblasts
Odontoblasts
Enamel
Dentine
Root sheath
Dental pulp

E. Mammary Glands

Mammary ridges
6th week
7th week
Primary bud
Secondary buds
4th month
Mammary pit
Lactiferous ducts
6th month
8th month
Position of accessory nipples

OVERVIEW

Integument, or skin, consists of 2 layers, the epidermis and dermis. The superficial epidermal layer develops from ectoderm. Hair follicles, sweat glands, sebaceous glands, and mammary glands all develop from epidermal projections into the dermis. The dermis is derived from mesoderm of the dermatomes as well as lateral plate mesoderm. Neural crest cells also contribute to dermis formation in the face and neck. Tooth development begins with the formation of ectodermal projections that become bell-shaped and wrap around mesenchyme derived from neural crest cells of the first pharyngeal arch. Tissue-tissue interactions between the dental bell and mesenchyme drive tooth formation. The ameloblasts (enamel-producing) are derived from the ectoderm, whereas the odontoblasts (dentin-producing), dental pulp, and cemento-blasts (cementum-producing) are derived from neural crest cells.

Epidermis

The integument, or skin, consists of 2 layers, the epidermis and dermis. The epidermis of the skin is derived from ectoderm and begins as a single layer of cells that eventually become stratified and organized into 3 layers: (1) the basal layer, (2) the intermediate layer, and (3) an outer squamous cell layer called *periderm* (**Part A**). The basal layer (stratum germinativum) contains the epidermal stem cells, which continually proliferate and are the source of replacement cells as cells are sloughed off. Some of the daughter cells in the basal layer differentiate into keratinocytes composing the intermediate layer of the epidermis. Progressive differentiation of the keratinocytes forms sublayers, including the inner stratum spinosum, stratum granulosum, and stratum corneum. The basal layer of the epidermis also is invaded by pigment cells (neural crest–derived melanocytes), Langerhans cells (immune cells), and Merkel cells (pressure-sensing cells). Portions of the epidermis, particularly on the surfaces of the fingertips, toes, hands, and feet, develop unique patterns of external projections or ridges (e.g., fingerprints) that are genetically determined.

Dermis

The dermis contains connective tissue, blood vessels, and muscle bundles and serves as a conduit for nerves. The dermis is derived from mesoderm of the dermatomes and lateral plate mesoderm. In the face and upper part of the neck, however, some of the dermis is derived from neural crest cells. As the dermis develops, 2 basic dermal layers arise. The papillary layer is more superficial and consists of projections of dermal mesoderm into the epidermis (dermal papillae) (**Part A**). Below this layer, the mesoderm forms a thick, dense, irregular connective tissue known as the *reticular layer*. Beneath the dermis, a fatty subcutaneous connective tissue layer, called the *hypodermis*, also forms from the mesoderm.

Hair

Hair follicles originate as solid epidermal projections penetrating the underlying dermis (**Part B**). These projections develop club-shaped shafts that become indented at the base by mesenchymal projections called the *dermal papillae of the hair*. Cells in the center of the shaft become keratinized, producing the hair shaft. The more peripheral (basal) cells of the shaft form the epithelial hair sheath, and at the base of the shaft, these cells form the germinal matrix. Cells of the germinal matrix continually proliferate and are responsible for the continued elongation of the hair shaft. A small smooth muscle, the arrector muscle of hair, forms within the nearby mesenchyme and becomes attached to the connective tissue surrounding the epithelial hair sheath. When this muscle contracts, it erects the hair. The first hair to appear is called *lanugo hair* and is usually shed and replaced by coarser hair.

Glands of the Skin

Sebaceous glands release an oily substance covering the hair and skin, and these glands develop from buds that branch off from the original epidermal hair bud (**Part B**). At birth, the outer epidermis is covered with a whitish paste called *vernix caseosa*. Vernix caseosa is a culmination of sebaceous gland secretions and dead epidermal cells, and the lanugo hair helps retain it on the outer skin surface. Vernix caseosa is thought to help protect the skin against the deleterious effects of prolonged exposure to amniotic fluid.

Sweat glands develop from epidermal buds growing into the underlying dermis (**Part C**). These buds form a long, coiled, unbranched solid shaft of epidermis that eventually canalizes. Cells of the deeper end of the shaft differentiate into secreting cells.

Teeth

Teeth develop from an ectodermal ridge forming on the oral surface of the maxillary and mandibular processes. Small ectodermal dental buds grow from this ridge into the underlying first pharyngeal arch mesenchyme, and each bud becomes bell-shaped (**Part D**). This bell-shaped dental cap encapsulates neural crest mesenchyme, forming the dental papillae. Dental cap cells adjacent to the dental papillae differentiate into ameloblasts (which deposit enamel). Cells of the dental papillae adjacent to the ameloblasts differentiate into odontoblasts (which deposit dentin). The cells of the dental papillae also form cementoblasts, which secrete cementum, the matrix anchoring the teeth to bone. Outside the dental organs, mesenchymal cells differentiate into bone and periodontal ligaments. As the roots of the dental papillae elongate, they push the teeth through the overlying soft tissue, causing them to erupt from beneath the epithelium within the first 2 years of life. The dental buds for permanent teeth form during the fetal period and do not usually erupt until about ages 5–7.

Mammary Glands

The mammary glands develop from epidermal thickenings called *mammary ridges* (**Part E**). Mammary ridges develop on both sides of the body along a line running from the axilla to the inguinal region. These ridges disappear except at the site of the breasts. Here, the primary epidermal buds grown down into the dermis as solid cords and branch. These cords eventually canalize and, by birth, form lactiferous ducts that open to the exterior surface at a depression called the *mammary pit*. The underlying mesenchyme surrounding this pit proliferates, forming a nipple that everts soon after birth. The epidermis immediately adjacent to the nipple forms the areola.

Anomalies

Atrichia is the congenital absence of hair. Hydrophilic ectodermal dysplasia is the absence of sweat glands and usually occurs as an X-linked trait. Affected infants are vulnerable to potentially lethal hyperpyrexia. Polythelia (supernumerary nipples) and polymastia (supernumerary breasts) are equally common in both sexes. In 1 in 2,000 births, teeth may be present at the time of birth. These natal teeth may be primary teeth that prematurely erupt or form as supernumerary teeth. Natal teeth can complicate breast-feeding and, if supernumerary, may interfere with the development of primary teeth.

40 The Fetal Period

A. Relative Proportions of Head & Body

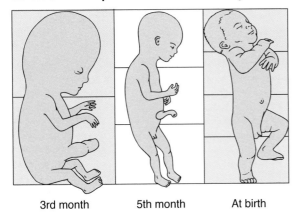

3rd month   5th month   At birth

B. Measurements for Gestational Age Determination

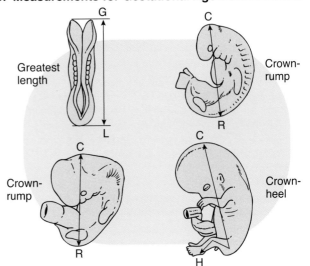

Greatest length

Crown-rump

Crown-rump

Crown-heel

C. Fetal Appearance

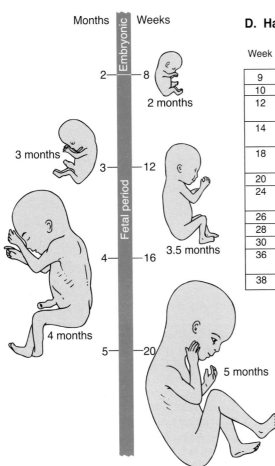

Months   Weeks

Embryonic

2 — 8

2 months

3 months

Fetal period

3 — 12

3.5 months

4 — 16

4 months

5 — 20

5 months

D. Hallmarks During the Fetal Period by Gestational Age

Week	Crown-Rump Length (mm)	Major Internal and External Characteristics
9	~50	Eyes closed. Ears low. Intestines within umbilical cord.
10	~61	Intestines in abdomen.
12	~87	Sex distinguishable externally. Primary ossification centers appear. Urine production is ongoing. Swallowing begins.
14	~120	Eyes face forward. Eye movement begins. Lower limbs well developed.
18	~160	Vernix caseosa covers the fetus. Fetal movements perceived by mother (quickening). Primordial ovarian follicles formed.
20	~190	Lanugo hair visible on head and body. Diurnal rhythms begin.
24	~230	Fingernails present. Alveolar type II cells differentiate and begin secreting surfactant.
26	~250	Lungs capable of breathing air. Eyes partially open.
28	~270	Eyes wide open. Subcutaneous fat deposition begins.
30	~280	Testes descending. Pupillary light reflex can be elicited.
36	~340	Body plump because of subcutaneous fat. Flexed limbs. Lanugo hair almost completely absent.
38	~360	Testes in scrotum or inguinal canal. Chest well developed.

E. Expected Date of Delivery (EDD)

	Days	Weeks	Lunar Months	Calendar Months
Fertilization	266	38	9.5	8.75
Last normal menstrual period (LNMP)	280	40	10.0	9.0

Nägele's rule for determining EDD: count back 3 months from the 1st day of the LNMP and add 1 year and 7 days. Example: if first day of LNMP was May 10, 2000, subtract 3 months (February 10, 2000) and add 1 year and 7 days (EDD = February 17, 2001). This is fairly accurate if the woman has a history of regular menstrual periods. Ultrasound measurements of crown-rump length can be used to better predict the gestational age.

OVERVIEW

The fetal period is the developmental period encompassing primarily the maturation of organs established during the embryonic period. Advances in diagnostic instrumentation and techniques permit the determination of gestational age, monitoring of development, detection of congenital anomalies, and even surgical repair of defects in utero. Viability of a newborn is its ability to survive outside the womb and is related to several factors, including gestational age at the time of birth and birth weight.

The Early Fetal Appearance

During the embryonic period, all of the major tissue and organ systems are established, and, for the most part, by the end of the eighth week all anatomical structures are easily recognizable. From this point forward, the period called the *fetal period*, body growth and tissue maturation are the main focus of development. At the beginning of the fetal period, the head is disproportionately large compared to the rest of the body; the head constitutes almost one half of the entire body length of the fetus (**Part A**). However, by midgestation this is reduced to a third, and, by the time of birth, the head constitutes only about one fourth of the entire body length. Diagnostic technology and surgical techniques have advanced to the point that certain life-threatening defects in the fetus can be repaired in utero, although such procedures remain very risky and experimental.

Trimesters of Pregnancy

The gestational period is generally divided into 3 trimesters, each 3 months long. The first trimester includes the entire embryonic period and early fetal period. By the end of the first trimester, all major organs have formed and are now beginning to mature (**Part B**). Primary ossification centers begin to show up, and the arms have almost reached their relative length (**Part C**). The external genitalia of the fetus have sufficiently developed so that the sex may be determined via ultrasound. The intestinal loops once occupying the umbilical cord have returned into the abdomen by the end of this period. Urine formation is ongoing, and urine is released into the amniotic fluid. Amniotic fluid is ingested and absorbed by the fetus's developing digestive system, and a portion of this absorbed fluid is transported into the maternal circulation via the placenta. Vascular circulation can be evaluated within 5 weeks into the first trimester using ultrasound. The embryonic heart rate is usually about 100 beats/min but increases to about 160 by 8 weeks and then drops to about 150 by the second trimester.

During the second trimester, the fetus grows and exhibits more anatomically distinguishable features (**Part C**). The bony skeleton is actively ossifying and is readily observed by ultrasound. By 17–18 weeks, fetal movements (called *quickening*) begin to be felt by the mother, and by 20–22 weeks, these fetal movements begin to show diurnal rhythms. Soon the testes begin their descent in male fetuses. Fat also begins to accumulate under the skin, and by the end of this trimester substantial weight gain begins. By 24 weeks, alveolar type II cells begin to differentiate and secrete surfactant. By the start of the third trimester, the fetus may survive if born prematurely, depending on the degree of maturity of the lungs, pulmonary circulation, and respiratory centers in the brain. By week 35, the fetus usually weighs at least 2,500 gm, and the respiratory and nervous systems are mature enough to sustain life outside the womb. By full term, the normal fetus weighs about 3,400 gm and has a crown-to-rump length of approximately 360 mm.

Estimating Embryonic and Fetal Age and Time of Birth

For the first 4 weeks of development, one can determine the age of an embryo by counting paraxial somites (about 3 pairs of somites/day beginning on day 20) and monitoring the external appearance of the pharyngeal arches. However, determining the developmental stage on this basis is difficult. Alternatively, an estimate of gestational age can be made by measuring the greatest length of the embryo using ultrasound (**Part D**). Once the cranial-caudal flexure becomes pronounced, gestational age is usually determined by measuring the crown-to-rump length during the first trimester. This straight-line measurement is the distance from the apex of the crown of the head to the apex of the rump and, again, is usually measured by ultrasonic imaging (usually accurate within 1 or 2 days). As the limbs develop, measuring the crown-to-heel length also provides a good estimate of gestational age. Fetal head (biparietal head diameter) and femur measurements can be used to refine this estimation even further during the second and third trimesters.

The date of birth is usually estimated from the date of onset of the last menstrual period (**Part E**). Although a patient may have regular menstrual cycles, the error of using this method for calculating gestational age ranges from 5% to 20%. Accuracy is greatly improved if the expected date of birth is calculated from the time of coitus during the ovulatory period, since fertilization usually occurs within 24 hours after ovulation (this date plus 266 days or 38 weeks). Regardless of the technique, birth usually occurs within 10–14 days of the calculated delivery date.

The usual gestational period is 266 days but can vary greatly. If the birth occurs well short of the 266 days, the baby is usually smaller and referred to as *premature*. Infants born well after the 266 days are referred to as *postmature* and have a higher risk of mortality for unknown reasons. Viability of the fetus is determined by its ability to survive outside the womb. Premature infants usually weigh between 1,500 and 2,500 gm; they are viable but usually present difficulties. Infants weighing < 500 gm at birth are usually not viable, but neonatal care and technology have increasingly lowered the mortality rates of these infants.

Abnormal Fetal Growth

There can be a large variation in the development rate, birth weight, and gestational age of newborns. *Intrauterine growth restriction* (IUGR) is a term applied to infants whose birth weight is in the lower 10th percentile for a given gestational age. Therefore, 1 in 10 infants suffers from IUGR. Such infants have an increased risk of neurological deficiencies and respiratory distress and a higher mortality rate. Large infants, on the other hand, also have an increased risk of mortality for reasons that are not understood. Causes of IUGR include poor maternal nutrition, smoking, multiple pregnancy, drug abuse (e.g., alcohol, cocaine), impaired uteroplacental blood flow (e.g., renal disease, hypotension), placental insufficiency (placental defect or infarct), and genetic factors (e.g., chromosomal aberrations such as Down syndrome). Low-weight babies, usually <2,500 gm, may be preterm infants (having a shortened gestation period) or full-term infants suffering from IUGR.

41 Fetal Membranes and Placenta I: Placental Structure

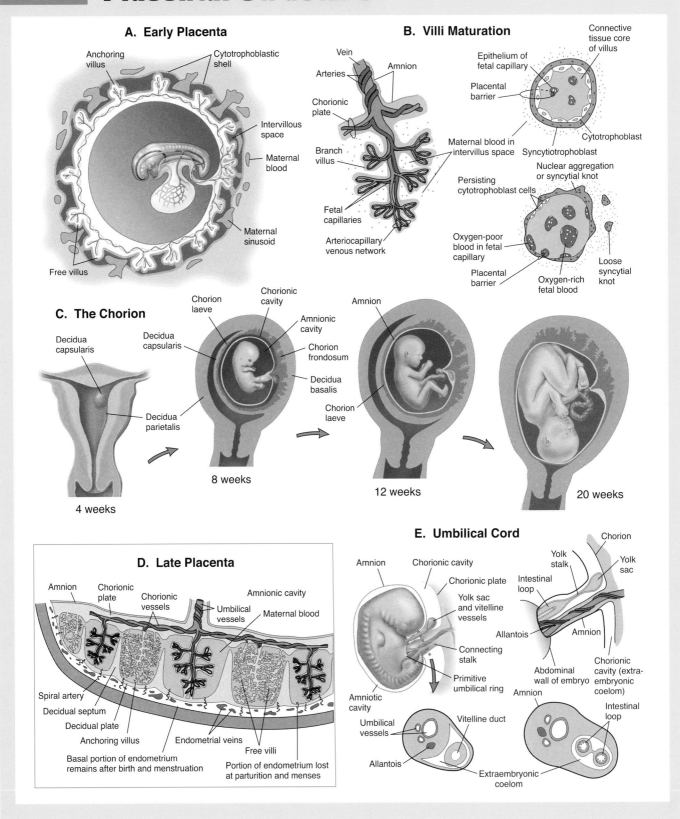

A. Early Placenta

Anchoring villus
Cytotrophoblastic shell
Intervillous space
Maternal blood
Maternal sinusoid
Free villus

B. Villi Maturation

Vein
Arteries
Amnion
Chorionic plate
Branch villus
Fetal capillaries
Arteriocapillary venous network
Maternal blood in intervillus space
Connective tissue core of villus
Epithelium of fetal capillary
Placental barrier
Cytotrophoblast
Syncytiotrophoblast
Nuclear aggregation or syncytial knot
Persisting cytotrophoblast cells
Oxygen-poor blood in fetal capillary
Placental barrier
Oxygen-rich fetal blood
Loose syncytial knot

C. The Chorion

Decidua capsularis
Decidua capsularis
Decidua parietalis
Chorion laeve
Chorionic cavity
Amnionic cavity
Chorion frondosum
Decidua basalis
Chorion laeve
Amnion

4 weeks
8 weeks
12 weeks
20 weeks

D. Late Placenta

Amnion
Chorionic plate
Chorionic vessels
Umbilical vessels
Amnionic cavity
Maternal blood
Spiral artery
Decidual septum
Decidual plate
Anchoring villus
Basal portion of endometrium remains after birth and menstruation
Endometrial veins
Free villi
Portion of endometrium lost at parturition and menses

E. Umbilical Cord

Amnion
Chorionic cavity
Chorionic plate
Yolk sac and vitelline vessels
Connecting stalk
Primitive umbilical ring
Amniotic cavity
Umbilical vessels
Allantois
Chorion
Yolk stalk
Yolk sac
Intestinal loop
Allantois
Amnion
Abdominal wall of embryo
Chorionic cavity (extra-embryonic coelom)
Amnion
Intestinal loop
Vitelline duct
Extraembryonic coelom

OVERVIEW

The placenta consists of the embryo-derived trophoblast (cytotrophoblasts and syncytiotrophoblasts) and chorionic plate and the maternally derived decidua basalis. The embryonic portion forms villous projections that protrude into syncytial-lined, maternal blood–filled sinuses. Some of these villi help anchor the chorionic plate to the decidua, whereas others project freely into the invervillous space and serve as the site of gaseous-nutrient exchange. The barrier between the maternal and fetal blood eventually is reduced to only a thin layer of syncytium and fetal endothelium. Implantation stimulates the endometrium to undergo a decidual reaction important for maintenance of the embryo and fetus. The umbilical cord functions to carry the blood vessels connecting the fetal and placental vasculature.

The Embryo/Fetal Portion

The trophoblast differentiates into 2 layers, the cytotrophoblastic and synctiotrophoblastic layers. As the trophoblast invades the endometrium, it penetrates maternal sinusoids, and maternal blood flows into the lacunar spaces within the syncytial layer. This establishes the early uteroplacental circulation. Here, oxygen, carbon dioxide, nutrients, and waste products are exchanged between the embryonic tissue and maternal blood by diffusion. To increase the surface area of the exchange, the lacunae expand, and cytotrophoblastic projections covered with syncytiotrophoblast cells protrude into the lacunae, forming villi. Eventually, the cores of these villi become populated by extraembryonic mesoderm and develop blood vessels that connect to those within the chorionic plate and primitive umbilicus (**Part A**). The chorionic plate is the extraembryonic mesoderm lining the extraembryonic coelom (chorionic cavity).

Some of the villi extend across the lacunae, and their cytotrophoblast cells penetrate the syncytial layer, attach to the endometrium, and form an outer cytotrophoblastic shell surrounding the implanting embryo (**Part A**). Because they extend from the chorionic plate to the cytotrophoblastic shell, these anchoring villi help secure the chorionic plate to the decidua. Other villi protrude into the lacunae of the intervillous space, forming free villi. Anchoring and free villi start out as primitive villi in that they have connective tissue separating the fetal capillaries from the cytotrophoblast and syncytium. However, after the fourth month, much of this connective tissue and many of the cytotrophoblasts disappear (**Part B**). In addition, the syncytium becomes thinner as some of the syncytial tissue breaks off into the intervillous space and enters the maternal circulation. These pieces are called *syncytial knots*. Eventually, the barrier between the maternal and fetal circulatory systems is reduced to a thin layer of syncytium and a fetal capillary endothelial cell.

The term *chorion* collectively refers to the trophoblast layer and chorionic plate. Early in development, villi cover the entire surface of the chorion, but development of the villi is more pronounced on the surface adjacent to the embryonic pole (chorion frondosum) (**Part C**). Elsewhere, the villi eventually degenerate, leaving a smooth chorionic surface (chorion laeve) that is noticeable by the eighth week.

Maternal Portion (Decidua)

The stroma of the endometrium undergoes a major transformation during implantation called the *decidua reaction*. The stromal cells enlarge and begin accumulating glycogen and lipids. Various designations are given to the different areas of the decidual endometrium depending on its relationship to the embryo or fetus (**Part C**). The endometrium opposite the chorion frondosum is called the *decidua basalis*. This part of the endometrial wall not occupied by the embryo is called the *decidua parietalis*. The endometrium overlying the fully implanted embryo is called the *decidua capsularis*. As the fetus increases in size, the decidua capsularis meets the decidua parietalis, and portions of the decidua capsularis disappear. Therefore, the chorion laeve comes in direct contact with the decidua parietalis,

obliterating the uterine cavity. In addition, fetal growth and increasing amniotic fluid levels cause the amnion to expand and fuse with the chorion, obliterating the chorionic cavity. Expansion of the uterine wall during pregnancy is driven primarily by hypertrophy of the uterine smooth muscle.

Placenta

The placenta consists of the decidual endometrium and chorion (**Part D**). The main functional region of the placenta consists of the chorion frondosum and the decidua basalis. The chorion increases in thickness at the expense of the decidua basalis. In areas where this expansion is less pronounced, the decidua develops projections called *decidual septa*. These septa separate the placenta into 15–20 compartments known as *cotyledons*. The placenta eventually covers approximately 15%–30% of the internal surface of the uterus, and at full term the placenta weighs approximately 500–600 gm. Eighty to 100 maternal spiral arteries penetrate the cytotrophoblastic shell and open into the intervillous spaces. Narrow openings at the ends of these arteries force blood deep into the spaces. As the pressure decreases, blood eventually makes its way back toward the decidua, entering endometrial veins. Collectively, the intervillous spaces hold about 150 mL of blood and are replenished 3–4 times/minute.

Umbilical Cord

The amnioectodermal junction is the junction between the amnion and the ectoderm found at the oval ring called the *primitive umbilical ring* (**Part E**). At 5 weeks, several structures pass through the ring: (1) the connecting stalk containing 2 umbilical arteries, 1 umbilical vein, and part of the allantois; (2) the vitelline duct (yolk stalk) and associated blood vessels; and (3) the canal connecting the intraembryonic and extraembryonic coelomic cavities. As the amniotic cavity enlarges and fuses with the chorionic plate, the amnion envelops the connecting stalk, vitelline duct, and coelomic space and crowds them together, forming the primitive umbilical cord. The intestinal loops withdraw back into the abdomen as the abdomen enlarges. Eventually, the vitelline duct, coelomic space, and distal allantois are obliterated. The yolk sac becomes trapped within the chorionic cavity and is obliterated. Ultimately, only the umbilical vessels remain within the cord, where they become surrounded by Wharton's jelly, an extracellular matrix that provides firm, yet flexible support for the umbilical cord.

The umbilical vessels usually join the chorionic vessels near the central point of the chorionic plate but may join them near the margin of the plate. If the cord inserts into the chorionic plate outside the placenta (velamentous insertion), the umbilical vessels are at high risk of tearing. Umbilical cord length usually ranges between 30 and 90 cm. It is tortuous and forms false knots (like twists in a telephone cord) and is about 1–2 cm in diameter. If the cord is exceedingly long, it can encircle the fetal neck or limbs, leading to strangulation or congenital defects. Restricted blood flow to the fetus, leading to fetal hypoxia, may result if the cord is compressed (prolapsed cord) between the fetus and the mother's bony pelvis.

A. Placental Transport

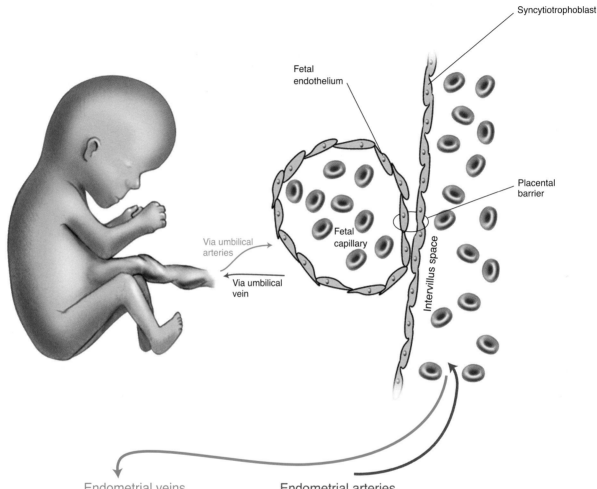

Syncytiotrophoblast

Fetal endothelium

Placental barrier

Fetal capillary

Intervillus space

Via umbilical arteries

Via umbilical vein

Endometrial veins

Waste products:
carbon dioxide, urea,
water, uric acid,
bilirubin

Other substances:
RBC antigens,
hormones

Endometrial arteries

Oxygen and nutrients:
water
carbohydrates
amino acids
lipids
electrolytes
hormones
vitamins
iron
trace elements

Harmful substances:
drugs (e.g. alcohol,
  heroin, cocaine)
poisons
carbon monoxide
viruses (e.g. rubella,
  cytomegalovirus, HIV)
strontium-90
toxoplasma gondii
diethylstilbestrol

Other substances:
antibodies
maternal lymphocytes

OVERVIEW

The placenta is one of the most metabolically active organs known, synthesizing huge amounts of protein and using almost one third of the oxygen and nutrients supplied to it for maintaining itself. The placenta is also an endocrine gland that secretes hormones, maintaining the corpus luteum and eventually taking over its function. All substances needed for maintaining the growth and development of the embryo and fetus are transported through the placenta, as are detrimental agents. Amniotic fluid serves to protect the fetus and allows fetal movement necessary for normal development. Abnormal fetal growth and development result if abnormally low or high levels of amniotic fluid exist.

Placental Metabolism

By 10 weeks, the placenta weighs about 50 gm and produces about 1.5 gm of protein/day. By term, it makes as much as 7.5 gm/day. No other organ, including the liver, synthesizes that much protein at that rate. Consequently, the placenta uses almost a third of all the oxygen and nutrients supplied to it for its own metabolism. The placenta synthesizes all of the glycogen, cholesterol, and fatty acids needed to fulfill the nutritional needs of itself as well as the fetus. Moreover, the placenta produces many hormones. Very early, the trophoblastic portion produces hCG, the hormone responsible for maintaining the corpus luteum past its usual 14-day life span in the menstrual cycle. By 4 months, the placenta produces enough progesterone and estrogen to maintain the pregnancy without the corpus luteum. Human chorionic somatomammotropin, a growth hormone–like substance synthesized by the placenta, gives the fetus priority for access to maternal blood glucose, making the mother somewhat diabetogenic.

Placental Exchange

Many substances are exchanged between the mother and the fetus through the placenta by diffusion, facilitated diffusion, active transport, and pinocytosis (**Part A**):

1. Oxygen, carbon dioxide, and carbon monoxide are exchanged. The fetus extracts up to 20–30 mL of oxygen/minute.
2. Nutrients and waste are exchanged, including amino acids, fatty acids, carbohydrates, vitamins, urea, bilirubin, uric acid, and others.
3. Many maternal antibodies are transported into the fetal capillaries, thereby providing passive immunity to various diseases. Maternal lymphocytes also cross into the fetal circulation. However, certain antibodies (e.g., against chicken pox and whooping cough) do not cross.
4. Most peptide hormones do not cross the placenta, but many unbound steroid hormones or synthetic hormones readily cross. Exposure of the fetus to diethylstilbestrol can lead to the formation of vaginal carcinomas and anomalous testis development in the offspring.
5. Infectious agents can pass through the placenta, including cytomegalovirus, rubella, measles, and syphilis bacteria. The human immunodeficiency virus (HIV) also can be transmitted through the placenta.
6. Most drugs easily cross, and many lead to cardiovascular and cerebral defects, lower birth rates, and high death rates. Drug addiction occurs in the fetus if the mother is using drugs such as heroin and cocaine. Teratogenic drugs include ethanol, cocaine, LSD, and heroin. Other teratogens crossing the placenta include excessive vitamin A, anticoagulants, antidepressive drugs, and chemotherapy drugs.

Near-Term Placenta

Several changes occur within the placenta near the end of gestation. Some of the capillaries within the villi become obliterated, and there is an increase in fibrous connective tissue and extracellular matrix that leads to an increase in villi thickness. There is also increased deposition of fibroid material between the decidua and fetal portion of the placenta, seemingly reducing placental function. Excessive fibroid formation can lead to infarction of intervillous spaces or whole cotyledons.

Amniotic Fluid

Amniotic fluid is a clear, watery fluid derived primarily from maternal blood and filling the amniotic cavity. Fluid levels increase from 30 to 350 mL between weeks 10 and 20, eventually reaching 800–1,000 mL by 37 weeks. The embryo and fetus are suspended in this liquid. The amniotic fluid functions (1) to absorb jolts, (2) to prevent embryo adhesion to the amnion, (3) to allow fetal movements, (4) to help maintain fetal body temperature, (5) as a barrier to infections, and (6) to permit symmetrical growth of the embryo. Amniotic fluid exchanges every 3 hours. Beginning as early as 12 weeks, the fetus begins swallowing the fluid, a portion of which is absorbed through the gut into the fetal bloodstream and ultimately passed into the maternal blood by way of the placenta. Occasionally, the amnion tears, forming amniotic bands (cords) that may encircle the fetus, particularly the limbs, leading to abnormal development of these structures or even amputations (1/1,200 live births).

Other Clinical Aspects

Abnormal levels of amniotic fluid can increase the risk of fetal or infant mortality or be indicative of certain congenital defects. *Hydramnios* and *polyhydramnios* are terms describing excessive amniotic fluid (1,500–2,000 mL and >2,000 mL, respectively). They may be due to idiopathic causes (35%), maternal diabetes (25%), or congenital anomalies that prevent the fetus from swallowing and transporting amniotic fluid (e.g., anencephaly and esophageal atresia). *Oligohydramnios* is the term describing low levels of amniotic fluid (< 400 mL). It may be caused by obstructive uropathy or fetal renal agenesis, in which case the fetus cannot excrete urine into the amniotic fluid. It also may be associated with premature rupture of the amnion. Premature rupture of the amnion with loss of amniotic fluid is the most common cause of premature labor.

43 Multiple Gestation Pregnancies

A. Dizygotic (Fraternal) Twins and Membranes

2 zygotes 2 cell stage Blastocyst stage Separate amnionic and chorionic sacs Separate placentas

1

Implantation of blastocysts

Fused chorionic sacs Fused placentas

2

Implantation of blastocysts close to each other

B. Monozygotic Twins by Division of Morula
(mechanism ∼ 35% of the time)

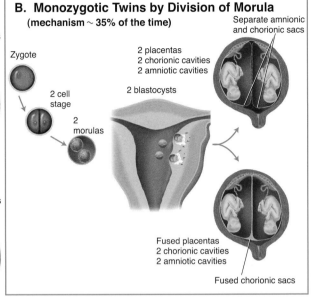

Zygote

2 cell stage

2 morulas

2 blastocysts

Separate amnionic and chorionic sacs

2 placentas
2 chorionic cavities
2 amniotic cavities

Fused placentas
2 chorionic cavities
2 amniotic cavities

Fused chorionic sacs

C. Monozygotic (Identical) Twins by Division of Inner Cell Mass (mechanism ∼ 65% of the time)

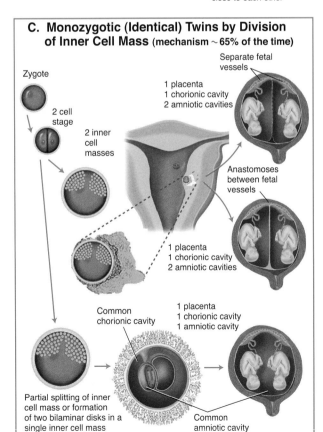

Zygote

2 cell stage

2 inner cell masses

Separate fetal vessels

1 placenta
1 chorionic cavity
2 amniotic cavities

Anastomoses between fetal vessels

1 placenta
1 chorionic cavity
2 amniotic cavities

Common chorionic cavity

1 placenta
1 chorionic cavity
1 amniotic cavity

Partial splitting of inner cell mass or formation of two bilaminar disks in a single inner cell mass

Common amniotic cavity

D. Classifications of Conjoined Twins

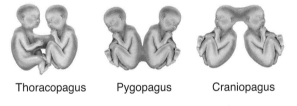

Thoracopagus   Pygopagus   Craniopagus

102

OVERVIEW

Infants from multiple gestation pregnancies have a higher risk of mortality and IUGR and are often born premature. Twins can result from the ovulation, fertilization, and implantation of two ova (dizygotic twins) or from the splitting of a single zygote, inner cell mass, or bilaminar disk (monozygotic twins). By examining the placental and fetal membranes, one can determine how the monozygotic twins were generated. Incomplete division of the inner cell mass or bilaminar disk can lead to the birth of conjoined twins, which are classified based on where the twins are joined.

Multiple Gestation Pregnancies

In the United States, about one in every 90 pregnancies results in twins and about 1 in 8,000 pregnancies results in triplets. The frequency of twinning is probably higher, but often one twin dies and is reabsorbed during development (sometimes called a vanishing twin). Multiple gestations of four or more are extremely rare but occur more frequently in women given fertility drugs. Twinning, particularly dizygotic twinning, also has a genetic tendency with the recurring risk being almost triple that of the general population. By studying monozygotic twins, we can investigate the interplay between the environment and genes in human development, pathology, and behavior.

Twinning and Fetal Membranes

Dizygotic (fraternal) twins are the most common type of twins, each infant having a different genotype. Dizygotic twins result from the ovulation and fertilization of 2 ova (**Part A**). Both blastocysts implant separately, developing their own placenta, chorion, and amnion. However, if they implant near each other, the placentas may fuse, and, if sufficiently intimate, each twin may share circulating RBCs (erythrocyte mosaicism).

Monozygotic (identical) twins have the same genotype, and any physical differences in monozygotic twins are environmentally induced. Monozygotic twins can form in two basic ways. A single fertilized zygote may split at the 2-cell stage (~35% of time), with each implanting separately and forming its own placenta, chorion, and amnion (**Part B**). More commonly, two inner cell masses form within a single blastula (~65% of time) (**Part C**). In this scenario, the twins share a common placenta and chorionic cavity but have separate amniotic cavities (monochorionic-diamniotic twins). Occasionally, monozygotic twins result from the splitting of a bilaminar disk, resulting in twins sharing a common placenta, chorion, and amnion (monochorionic-monoamniotic twins).

Clinical Aspects

Multiple gestation pregancies are high-risk pregnancies with mortality rates greater than single births. There also is the risk of premature birth and IUGR in multiple birth pregnancies. Mortality rates can reach as high as 60–100% for both twins in cases of twin transfusion syndrome. This syndrome is commonly seen in monochorionic-diamniotic twins, when arterial blood from one twin is shunted into the venous circulation of the other twin through a placental arteriovenous shunt. The result is that the donor twin is usually smaller and anemic, while the recipient twin is larger and polycythemic.

When monozygotic twins are generated from a split bilaminar disk and the disks are very close to one another, there may be incomplete separation of the twins. This results in the formation of conjoined twins. Conjoined twins are generally classified based on the axial level of the connection (thoracopagus, pygopagus, and carniopagus) (**Part D**). Many conjoined twins have been successfully separated through surgery. A parasitic twin is a conjoined twin whereby a very normal-looking portion of a body protrudes from an otherwise normal host twin.

In approximately 0.1–0.5% of pregnancies, the inner cell mass of a blastula does not develop properly so that a portion or entire embryo is missing. These are molar pregnancies. Levels of hCG hormone become abnormally high, the menstrual cycle is halted, and very little chorionic vasculature is present. A partial mole contains some embryonic tissue or an abnormal fetus that is triploidy and usually aborted in the second trimester. With a complete mole, there is no embryonic tissue. Tissue from molar pregnancies needs to be removed because residual trophoblastic tissue leads to formation of tumors. Tumors from partial molar pregnancies are usually benign, whereas tumors from a complete mole usually become malignant (choriocarcinomas).

Parturition and Changes in Fetal Circulation

A. Stages of Labor

Dilatation stage

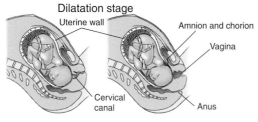

Uterine wall
Amnion and chorion
Vagina
Cervical canal
Anus

Expulsion stage

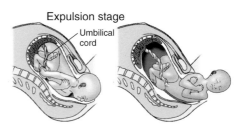

Umbilical cord

Placental stage

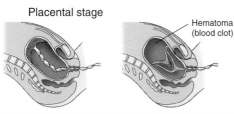

Hematoma (blood clot)

Recovery stage

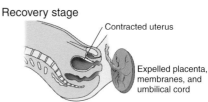

Contracted uterus
Expelled placenta, membranes, and umbilical cord

B. Fetal Circulation and Changes at Birth

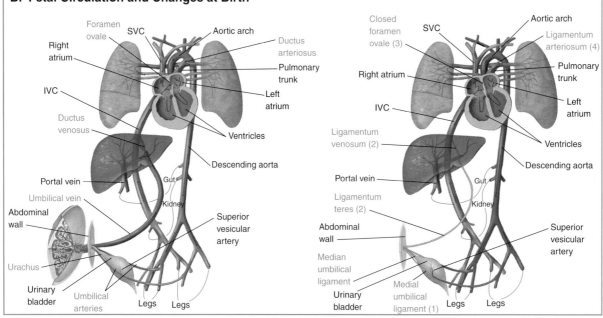

Foramen ovale
SVC
Aortic arch
Right atrium
Ductus arteriosus
Pulmonary trunk
IVC
Left atrium
Ductus venosus
Ventricles
Descending aorta
Portal vein
Gut
Kidney
Umbilical vein
Abdominal wall
Superior vesicular artery
Urachus
Urinary bladder
Umbilical arteries
Legs
Legs

Closed foramen ovale (3)
SVC
Aortic arch
Ligamentum arteriosum (4)
Right atrium
Pulmonary trunk
IVC
Left atrium
Ligamentum venosum (2)
Ventricles
Descending aorta
Portal vein
Gut
Kidney
Ligamentum teres (2)
Abdominal wall
Superior vesicular artery
Median umbilical ligament
Urinary bladder
Medial umbilical ligament (1)
Legs
Legs

C. Prenatal Hemolytic Disease

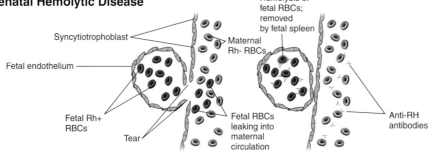

Syncytiotrophoblast
Fetal endothelium
Fetal Rh+ RBCs
Tear
Hemolysis of fetal RBCs; removed by fetal spleen
Maternal Rh- RBCs
Fetal RBCs leaking into maternal circulation
Anti-RH antibodies

Immunization of mother with fetal Rh+ RBCs   Presence of maternal Anti-Rh antibodies

OVERVIEW

Parturition is the process of childbirth, and labor is the term for the uterine contractions leading to delivery of the fetus and expulsion of the placenta. There are 4 basic stages of labor: (1) dilatation of the cervix, (2) expulsion of the fetus, (3) expulsion of the placenta, and (4) uterine contractions restricting blood flow from the uterine arteries that once supplied the placenta. Several circulatory adaptations found in the fetus no longer function in the newborn and adult. These modifications were used to increase efficient delivery of oxygen and nutrients to fetal tissues during development. After birth, these modifications regress or become nonfunctional.

Stages of Labor

Parturition is the process of childbirth and occurs in several stages. Parturition includes expulsion of the fetus, placenta, and fetal membranes (**Part A**). *Labor* is the term for the involuntary uterine contractions dilating the cervix and expelling the fetus and placenta.

1. The dilatation stage progressively widens the cervical opening. It begins with painful contractions of the uterus that are <10 minutes apart. It is usually the longest stage.
2. The expulsion stage is when the baby passes through the cervix and vagina and is delivered. The period for this stage usually ranges from 20 to 60 minutes.
3. The placental stage begins after delivery of the baby. During this stage, the placenta and fetal membranes are expelled through a series of uterine contractions lasting 15–30 minutes.
4. The recovery period is the final stage and lasts about 2 hours. During the stage, the myometrium continually contracts, helping to constrict the spiral arteries that previously supplied the placenta.

The mechanisms triggering parturition are poorly understood. Oxytocin can stimulate uterine contractions and is used clinically to induce labor. Evidence suggests that fetal factors may play a larger role than maternal factors in initiating parturition.

Fetal Circulation and Changes at Birth

Several adaptations in the fetal circulation increase the effective transport and delivery of oxygen- and nutrient-enriched blood to the fetal tissues. The developing fetus lives submerged in amniotic fluid but still needs a supply of oxygen and nutrients and needs to eliminate wastes. As far as the fetus is concerned, the placenta serves as its lung, GI tract, and kidney. For the exchange of carbon dioxide, oxygen, nutrients, and wastes, the fetus develops an additional set of blood vessels, the umbilical arteries (paired) and the umbilical vein. These vessels connect the fetus to the placental vasculature where the exchange occurs. In addition, the fetus develops vascular shunts so that the bulk of the blood flow bypasses the fetal lungs (via the ductus arteriosus and foramen ovale) and liver (via the ductus venosus) (**Part B**). Oxygen-rich blood enters the fetus via the umbilical vein and mixes with less saturated blood in the fetus. Mixing of desaturated with saturated blood occurs at several points (see left diagram of **Part B**):

1. At the junction of the ductus venosus and hepatic portal veins.
2. At the junction of the ductus venosus and inferior vena cava.
3. In the right atrium where the umbilical venous blood mixes with blood from the superior vena cava.
4. In the left atrium where blood passing through the foramen ovale mixes with deoxygenated blood returning from the pulmonary veins.
5. At the site of ductus arteriosus–aorta junction, where the less oxygenated blood of the pulmonary artery (less oxygenated because of prior mixing with superior vena caval blood in the right atrium) re-enters the aorta.

Several changes in the fetal circulation occur at birth with the cessation of placental blood flow and beginning of respiration (see numbers in right diagram of **Part B**):

1. The distal portion of the umbilical arteries contracts and closes within minutes. These vessels are obliterated at the distal ends, forming the medial umbilical ligaments, but their proximal ends become the superior vesical arteries supplying the bladder.
2. The umbilical vein and ductus venosus contract, close, and are obliterated, forming the ligamentum teres hepatis and ligamentum venosum, respectively.
3. Functional closure of the foramen ovale occurs as a result of decreased right atrial pressure and increased left atrial pressure (resulting from inflation of the lungs and a decrease in pulmonary resistance). With these pressure changes, septum primum is pushed against septum secundum even during diastole. Usually these septa seal shut within a year.
4. Closure of the ductus arteriosus usually occurs within 1–15 hours and forms the ligamentum arteriosum.

Clinical Aspects

Congenital torticollis (wryneck) is a fixed rotation and tilting of the head because of fibrosis and shortening of the sternocleidomastoid muscle. It can occur as a consequence of injury to this muscle during birth. However, it has been observed in a few cesarean births, suggesting additional etiologies.

Small amounts of fetal blood may enter the maternal circulation through small tears at the villi surface (**Part C**). If the fetus has Rh-positive blood and the mother is Rh-negative, a maternal immune response may be elicited. Anti-Rh antibodies cross the placenta, causing hemolysis of fetal RBCs and, in some cases, if severe enough, leading to anemia and prenatal hemolytic disease (erythroblastosis fetalis). The fetus may die unless delivered early or given an intrauterine blood transfusion of Rh-negative blood. The severity of the disease is more acute in pregnancies following an earlier birth of an Rh-positive infant (mixing of blood and immunization occur at parturition). Much of the hemoglobin released by the ruptured fetal RBCs is metabolized into bilirubin and removed by the maternal liver. However, after birth, jaundice may appear in these newborns because their livers may not be able to remove the large amounts of remaining bilirubin. As a consequence of the anemia, the liver and spleen may enlarge (sites of fetal hematopoeisis), and immature nucleated RBCs may be present in the circulation. The incidence of prenatal hemolytic disease has decreased with the introduction of Rh immunoglobulin treatment in Rh-negative mothers after the birth of Rh-positive infants.

Severe consequences can result if the normal circulatory modifications after birth are incomplete or fail. Patent ductus arteriosus and patent foramen ovale are common and are discussed in Chapters 32–35.

45 | Prenatal Diagnosis

A. Techniques for Prenatal Diagnosis

	CVS	*Amniocentesis*	*P UBS*
Gestational age performed	10–12 wks	16–18 wks	> 18 wks
Risk of miscarriage	0.5%	0.5%	1%
Benefits of screening	Early diagnosis	Relative safety	Provides blood sample for hematological studies

B. Prenatal Diagnosis by Amniocentesis

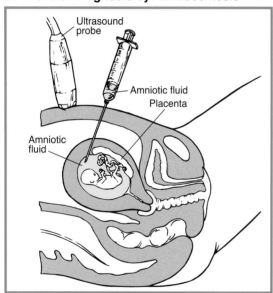

C. Prenatal Diagnosis by CVS

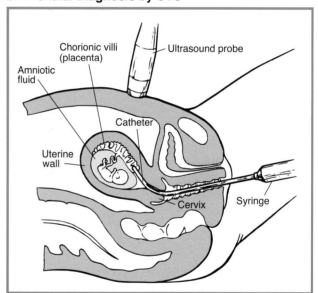

D. Prenatal Diagnosis by PUBS

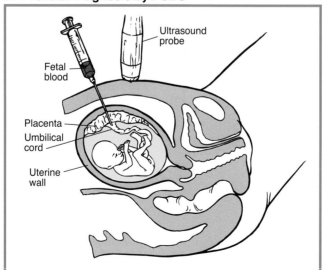

*From *Quick Look Genetics*, by Patricia Hoffer, 1999, with permission of Fence Creek Publishing, Inc. Madison, CT.

OVERVIEW

Advances in prenatal diagnosis have reduced the rates of perinatal mortality by enabling parents to make informed decisions that lower the risks to their child and improve their child's well-being. Prenatal monitoring can reduce the frequency or severity of genetic and congenital diseases by: (1) identifying parents who are potential carriers of genetic diseases and counseling them before their first pregnancy; (2) identifying fetal disorders early in the pregnancy, permitting therapeutic interventions that are necessary before the birth of the child; and (3) screening newborns for disorders and implementing preventive treatments before the onset of symptoms.

Indications for Prenatal Diagnosis

Perinatology is the area of medicine concerned with the health of the fetus and newborn. Prenatal diagnostic procedures are used to determine whether a fetus may have congenital defects or be at risk for a genetic disorder. Only at-risk pregnancies should be subjected to prenatal diagnosis because an increased risk of miscarriage accompanies these tests. Unfortunately, not all at-risk pregnancies can be identified. Indicators supporting the use of perinatal diagnostic include: (1) maternal age of 35 years or older; (2) the birth of a previous child with trisomy; (3) the birth of a previous child with congenital defects; (4) the birth of a previous child with a metabolic disorder; (5) parents in a high-risk group for a particular inherited disorder; (6) the presence of a chromosome abnormality in either parent; and (7) the presence of abnormal biochemical markers in maternal serum or amniotic fluid (e.g., α-fetoprotein).

Ultrasonography

In ultrasonography, ultra-high frequencies of sound are used to produce images of the placenta and fetus. Ultrasound is noninvasive, making it one of the most common prenatal diagnostic tools used in the United States. Moreover, the technology has advanced to the point that one can not only determine fetal age, placental size, and placental position but also image fetal blood flow, guide needles and catheters, and detect several congenital anomalies.

Amniocentesis

Sampling of fluid from the amniotic cavity is referred to as amniocentesis. Ultrasound is used to position a needle into the amniotic cavity, and about 20–30 mL of amniotic fluid is removed (**Part A**). Fetal cells in the fluid are usually cultured for 2–3 weeks and then used for cytogenetic analysis. Polymerase chain reaction (PCR) analysis is now used to assess particular genetic traits or mutations. PCR can be performed without the need for culturing the cells so that results from tests can be obtained much more quickly. The amniotic fluid can also be analyzed for the presence of particular proteins or metabolic products. Amniocentesis is usually performed after 16 weeks of gestation. Although fetal injury is rarely a problem, there is an increased risk of spontaneous abortion (1/200).

Chorionic Villi Sampling (CVS)

In chorionic villi biopsies, a catheter is passed through the cervix or maternal abdomen, and a small piece of villi tissue (10–40 mg) is aspirated by needle biopsy (**Part B**). Again, ultrasonography plays a key role in guiding the placement of the catheter and needle. Because villi have the same origin as the fetus, this tissue provides the same cytogenetic and biochemical information as found in cells obtained by amniocentesis. Because the procedure can be performed much earlier in pregnancy (i.e., 9–10 weeks of gestation), test results can be obtained ealier in the gestational period. One disadvantage of this technique is the 1% failure rate in obtaining a sample, and care must be taken not to sample maternal tissue. The risk of spontaneous abortion is similar to aminocentesis; thus, the need for a chorionic villi biopsy must be warranted.

Percutaneous Umbilical Blood Sampling

Percutaneous umbilical blood sampling is used to obtain fetal blood samples or to deliver medications to the fetus (**Part C**). It can be performed as early as 18 weeks of gestation. In this procedure, a needle is guided into the umbilical vein of the umbilical cord with the aid of ultrasonography. Blood samples obtained in this manner can be used for chromosomal analysis or biochemical diagnoses. Because the risk of miscarriage or fetal death is approximately 1%, this technique is usually not used for diagnostic procedures. Rather, it is used to treat fetal infections, deliver medications, or perform fetal blood transfusions (e.g., in severe cases of prenatal hemolytic disease).

Interventions

Because of advancements in prenatal diagnosis and surgical techniques, it is becoming increasingly possible to perform corrective surgery on the fetus while in the uterus. Intrauterine corrective surgery, although still very risky, has been performed successfully for such anomalies as diaphragmatic hernias, hydrocephaly involving stenosis of the aqueduct of Sylvius, and obstructive uropathy. The potential to treat genetic orders in which a single gene product is missing or abnormal lies in gene therapy. In gene therapy, the normal version of the gene must be stably integrated into the genome of the patient's cells. Once the gene is integrated, its expression must be properly regulated and its product synthesized in sufficient quantities to alleviate symptoms of the disease. Although gene therapy is very much in its infancy and highly experimental, success has been achieved in several animal models. Experimental trials using gene therapy to treat several human inherited disease are now ongoing. These diseases include Gaucher's disease, adenosine deaminase deficiency, familial hypercholesterolemia, Duchenne muscular dystrophy, and autoimmune rheumatoid arthritis.

A. Causes of Birth Defects

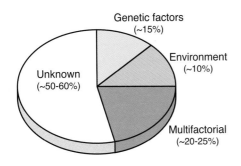

Genetic factors (~15%)

Environment (~10%)

Unknown (~50-60%)

Multifactorial (~20-25%)

B. General Susceptibility

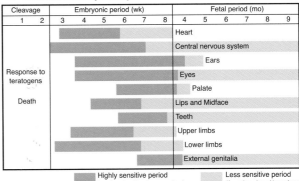

Cleavage	Embryonic period (wk)	Fetal period (mo)
1 2	3 4 5 6 7 8	4 5 6 7 8 9

Response to teratogens

Death

Heart
Central nervous system
Ears
Eyes
Palate
Lips and Midface
Teeth
Upper limbs
Lower limbs
External genitalia

■ Highly sensitive period (major structural anomalies)   ■ Less sensitive period (functional and/or minor structural anomalies)

C. Examples of Known Teratogens

	Agent	Associated Congenital Defects
Infections	Cytomegalovirus	Microcephaly, blindness, mental impairment
	Rubella virus	Cataracts, glaucoma, heart defects, deafness
	HIV	Microcephaly
	Toxoplasma gondii	Hydrocephalus, microphthalmia
	Treponema pallidum	Mental impairment, deafness
	Herpes simplex virus	Microphthalmia, microcephaly, retinal dysplasia
Drugs	Alcohol	Fetal alcohol syndrome, mental impairment, heart defects, craniofacial anomalies
	Angiotensin-converting enzyme Inhibitors	IUGR, oligohydraminios, calvarial bone hypoplasia, renal dysfunction, fetal death
	Valproic acid	Neural tube, heart, and craniofacial defects, limb anomalies
	Warfarin	Chondrodysplasias, microcephaly, mental impairment, eye anomalies
	Thalidomide	Limb and heart defects
	Lithium	Heart and great-vessel defects
	Cocaine	IUGR, microcephaly, urogenital defects, neurobehavioral disorders
	Trimethadione	IUGR, craniofacial, heart, and limb defects, urogenital anomalies
	Retinoic acid (vitamin A)	Craniofacial, heart, neural tube, and limb defects
	Diethylstilbestrol	Abnormalities in uterus, uterine tubes, and vagina
	Nicotine	IUGR
Environmental Chemicals	Lead and mercury	IUGR, neurological disorders
	Polychlorinated biphenyls (PCBs)	IUGR, skin anomalies
Radiation		Microcephaly, mental impairment, skeletal anomalies, IUGR, cataracts, NTDs
Maternal factors	Diabetes mellitus	Varies but commonly includes hydramnios and heart and neural tube defects

D. Examples of Genetic Disorders

	Genetic Anomaly	Phenotype
Chromosomal Number	Trisomy 21 (Down syndrome)	Mental impairment, characteristic facial appearance, prominent palmar crease, increased risk of heart and craniofacial defects
	Trisomy 18 (Edward's syndrome)	Severe IUGR, craniofacial anomalies, clenched fists, rocker-bottom feet, cardiac and renal anomalies
	Trisomy 13 (Patau syndrome)	Incomplete development of forebrain and optic nerves, major craniofacial anomalies, heart and renal defects, omphalocele, and polydactyly
	Klinefelter's syndrome (XXY)	Sterile, testicular atrophy, often gynecomastia (enlarged breasts)
	Turner's syndrome (XO)	Ovaries absent, webbed neck, lymphedema of limbs, skeletal anomalies, and mental impairment
Chromosomal Structural Anomalies	Translocations	Trisomy and deletions of chromosomal segments, responsible for a subgroup of Down syndrome
	Deletions	Cri du chat, del[5][p15.5] Smith-Magensis syndrome, del[17][p11.2] Catch-22 syndrome, del[22][q11] DiGeorge syndrome, del[22][q11.2]
	Microdeletions	Prader-Willi syndrome, del[15][q11-q13] paternal origin Angelman syndrome, del[15][q11-q13] maternal origin
Mutations	Fibroblast growth factor-3 receptor	Achondroplasia
	FMRI gene	Fragile X syndrome
	CFTR gene	Cystic fibrosis
	Hexokinase A and glucocerebrosidase	Tay-Sachs and Gaucher disease, respectively
	Phenylalanine hydroxylase	Phenylketonuria
	pRB gene	Retinoblastoma
	Dystrophin	Duchenne muscular dystrophy
	Low-density-lipoprotein receptor	Familial hypercholesterolemia
	Clotting factor enzymes	Hemophilia
	Guanosine triphospatase	Neurofibromatosis type 1
	Hemoglobin α and β	Thalassemia α and β

E. Types of Chromosomal Structural Errors

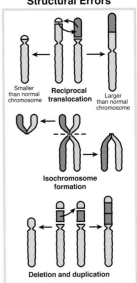

Smaller than normal chromosome   **Reciprocal translocation**   Larger than normal chromosome

Isochromosome formation

Deletion and duplication

OVERVIEW

Teratology is the study of the causes of congenital anomalies. Fifty-sixty percent of congenital defects are of unknown etiology. The remaining cases are due to genetic factors, environmental factors, and multifactorial inheritance. Several environmental factors as well as teratogenic agents have been identified: (1) exposure to drugs, (2) exposure to infectious agents, (3) exposure to environmental chemicals, (4) exposure to radiation, and (5) nutritional deficiencies. Known genetic factors causing defects include (1) nondisjunction events, (2) chromosomal aberrations, and (3) gene mutations.

Teratology

Teratology is the science of studying the causes of congenital anomalies (birth defects). Major structural anomalies occur in 5%–6% of the population, and congenital defects are the leading cause of mortality in infants and a major contributor to disabilities. Congenital anomalies are due to genetic factors (~15%), environmental factors (10%), and a combination of genetic and environmental factors (multifactorial inheritance, ~20%–25%) (**Part A**). Unfortunately, 50%–60% of the birth defects have an unknown etiology, and most originate during the embryonic period. Varying terms are used to describe congenital anomalies:

1. *Malformations* are defects resulting from complete absence of a structure or from alteration in its normal development.
2. *Disruptions* are destructive or interfering processes leading to abnormal development (e.g., vascular accidents).
3. *Deformations* are alterations in structure due to improper mechanical forces molding a part of the fetus over a prolonged period of time (e.g., amputation of a limb due to amniotic banding).
4. *Dysplasias* are abnormal tissue amounts or organization leading to abnormal development.

The term *syndrome* refers to a group of anomalies that occur together and that usually have a common etiological origin. The term *association* refers to the coincident appearance of 2 or more anomalies that occur more frequently together than would be expected by chance alone but whose etiological basis is unknown.

Environmental Factors

Environmental agents recognized as causing or increasing the risk of congenital defects upon maternal exposure are called *teratogens*. Exposure to these agents and the developmental events that they perturb may occur well before the consequences manifest themselves morphologically or physiologically. Various organs and tissues have different critical periods of development. Therefore, not only is the exposure level of a teratogenic agent important but so are the timing and the duration of exposure (**Part B**). Perturbation in development before the beginning of the embryonic period usually results in spontaneous abortion, whereas perturbation during the embryonic period can cause major morphological anomalies that may not be fatal or a major handicap in utero. In the fetal period, most organ systems are already established, and further development primarily involves growth and maturation. Exposure to teratogenic agents during the fetal period, therefore, may result in less obvious morphological defects but be physiologically substantial (i.e., brain maturation). Identifiable agents cause only about 10% of congenital anomalies, but new agents are being continually identified. Environmental agents known to increase the risk of congenital defects can be divided into several categories (**Part C**):

1. Infectious agents. Certain microorganisms and viruses cross the placenta and infect the embryo and fetus, leading to congenital defects. Some are listed in **Part C**.

2. Drugs. Maternal exposure to particular drugs can cause congenital defects or anomalies. Alcohol consumed during pregnancy is a significant teratogen. Fetal alcohol syndrome occurs at rate of 0.1%–0.2% of live births and may be the most common cause of behavioral and learning disabilities in children. Cigarette smoking causes IUGR, therefore increasing the risk of infant death. Other teratogenic agents are listed in **Part C**.
3. Environmental chemicals. Maternal exposure to environmental pollutants or exposure to industrial and agricultural chemicals may be teratogenic.
4. Radiation. Exposure to ionizing radiation during the embryonic period can lead to spontaneous abortion or anomalies ranging from IUGR to major congenital anomalies.
5. Nutritional insufficiencies. Supplementation of the diet with folic acid significantly reduces the risk of NTDs. Vitamin A deficiency or excess is also teratogenic.

Genetic Factors

Genetic factors may cause one third of all congenital anomalies. Those known to be based on genetic factors can be broken down into 3 main categories (**Part C**):

1. Abnormal chromosome number. Abnormal chromosome number usually results from nondisjunction of chromosomes during gametogenesis. Nondisjunction involves either autosomes or sex chromosomes. Aneuploidy occurs when an individual has an abnormal chromosome number for any particular chromosome set. In monosomy, the individual only has 1 parental representative but not both. Most monosomies are not viable, with the exception of Turner's syndrome. In trisomy, the individual has 1 chromosome from 1 parent and 2 from the other. Many trisomies do survive, the most common one being trisomy 21 (Down syndrome).
2. Chromosomal aberrations (**Part E**). Chromosomal aberrations usually result from chromosomal breakage followed by abnormal recombination. Translocation is the transfer of a piece of 1 chromosome onto a nonhomologous chromosome. While it may not affect embryological development, future germ cells produced by this individual will be abnormal. Chromosomal deletions can result from a chromosomal break with subsequent loss of that piece. An example is cri du chat syndrome, in which the short arm of chromosome 5 is deleted. Microdeletions (i.e., deletions removing just a few genes rather than large pieces of chromosomes) have been increasingly recognized as technology permits higher-resolution analysis of the human genome. Abnormal development also can occur if a portion of a chromosome is duplicated.
3. Mutations. About 8% of congenital anomalies involve mutations in specific genes. These mutations usually lead to a loss or change in function of a gene product. Anomalies caused by mutant genes are inherited according to Mendelian laws; therefore, the likelihood of affecting the child of a couple can be predicted and tested using prenatal diagnostic procedures.

For each of the following questions, choose the **one best answer**.

1. A breathing newborn exhibits severe cyanosis immediately after birth and dies. Autopsy results show that both ventricles were of normal size and there was no evidence of an atrial or ventricular septal defect. Moreover, the lungs were of normal size and well inflated. What is the most likely diagnosis?

(A) Tetralogy of Fallot

(B) Transposition of the great vessels

(C) Aortic valvular stenosis

(D) Pulmonary valvular atresia

(E) Patent ductus arteriosus

2. During dissection of a cadaver, you notice that there is a ligamentous structure connecting the aortic arch and the pulmonary artery. A plexus of nerves covers it, and a branch of the vagus nerve apparently runs beneath this ligament and back up into the neck. What is the embryological origin of this ligamentous structure?

(A) It is a remnant of the right third aortic arch.

(B) It is remnant of the left fourth aortic arch.

(C) It is a remnant of the right sixth aortic arch.

(D) It is a remnant of the left sixth aortic arch.

(E) It is a remnant of the left umbilical vein.

3. A newborn exhibits severe cyanotic symptoms in the abdomen, pelvis, and lower limbs but not in the head and neck or upper limbs. What is the most likely explanation?

(A) This child has a preductal coarctation of the aorta.

(B) This child has a postductal coarctation of the aorta.

(C) This child has a patent ductus arteriosus.

(D) This child has transposition of the great vessels.

(E) This child has a right aortic arch.

Questions 4 and 5.
While dissecting a cadaver, you find a fibrous cord within a fold of peritoneum running from the navel to the liver.

4. What is the embryological origin of this structure?

(A) The umbilical artery

(B) The right umbilical vein

(C) The left umbilical vein

(D) The subcardinal vein

(E) The urachus

5. Upon further dissection you find another fibrous cord within the liver spanning between the hepatic vein and the cord described above. What is this structure?

(A) The ligamentum teres hepatis

(B) The ligamentum venosum

(C) The ligamentum arteriosum

(D) A remnant of the right supracardinal vein

(E) The hepatogastric ligament

6. A newborn has a hypoplastic right ventricle, hypertrophic left ventricle, and patent foramen ovale. What is your initial diagnosis?

(A) Tricuspid atresia

(B) Pulmonary valvular stenosis

(C) Ostium primum defect

(D) Tetralogy of Fallot

(E) Aortic valvular atresia

7. A newborn with a cleft lip and cleft palate is cyanotic, and Doppler ultrasonic imaging reveals reduced pulmonary blood flow and a VSD. An electrocardiogram also suggests the presence of right ventricular hypertrophy. What is the most likely diagnosis?

(A) Transposition of the great vessels

(B) Tetralogy of Fallot

(C) Wolff-Parkinson-White syndrome

(D) Ostium secundum defect

(E) Aortic valvular atresia

8. Which of the following represents the correct temporal sequence for the appearance of hematopoietic sites during development?

(A) Chorionic mesoderm → liver → bone marrow → spleen

(B) Intraembryonic mesoderm → liver → bone marrow

(C) Yolk sac mesoderm → liver → spleen → bone marrow

(D) Yolk sac mesoderm → intraembryonic mesoderm → liver → bone marrow

(E) Precardiac mesoderm → liver → spleen → bone marrow

9. A set of twins is born, and upon examination of the fetal and placental membranes you find a single placenta with 2 amniotic cavities. What is the most likely scenario that led to the formation of these twins?

(A) Two ova were fertilized.

(B) The zygote split at the 2-cell stage.

(C) The blastula formed 2 separate inner cell masses.

(D) The blastula generated a single inner cell mass that subsequently formed 2 bilaminar disks.

(E) A single ovum was fertilized by 2 spermatozoa.

10. You deliver a newborn baby that appears normal, but almost a year later you see that the infant is beginning to show signs of cyanosis. Closer inspection shows that the right ventricle has hypertrophied and there are signs of pulmonary congestion and edema.

Auscultation of the heart and subsequent ultrasound tests indicate that all the valves appear to be normal. Which one of the following congenital heart defects is most likely responsible for the symptoms?

(A) Tetralogy of Fallot

(B) Transposition of the great vessels

(C) VSD

(D) Common atrioventricular canal

(E) Double superior vena cava

11. A 30-year-old pregnant woman has a large weight gain, and ultrasound suggests that there is more amniotic fluid than normal. Amniocentesis sampling showed an elevated α-fetoprotein level in the amniotic fluid. What is the most likely diagnosis?

(A) Polyhydramnios caused by esophageal atresia

(B) Oligohydramnios caused by fetal renal agenesis

(C) Amniotic banding syndrome

(D) Oligohydramnios with hypospadias

(E) Polyhydramnios caused by anencephaly

12. A 30-year-old woman gives birth to a second child that rapidly developed jaundice. The baby's liver and spleen were enlarged, and a blood sample revealed the presence of nucleated RBCs. What is one possible explanation?

(A) Both children were Rh-negative and the mother was Rh-positive.

(B) Both children were Rh-positive and the mother was Rh-negative.

(C) There was a partial detachment of the placenta during gestation.

(D) There was a congenital absence of the thymus in the second child.

(E) Hematopoiesis continued within the liver and was not transferred to the bone marrow in the second child.

13. As a physician, you want to better estimate the gestational age of the fetus because the pregnancy is high risk and may require an early delivery. Which of the following would you use to assess fetal age during the third trimester?

(A) Greatest length

(B) Crown-rump length

(C) Somite number

(D) Placental size

(E) Fetal heart rate

14. The risk of delivering a full-term, low-birth-weight baby increases as a consequence of all of the following except:

(A) Cigarette smoking by the mother

(B) Being part of a multiple birth

(C) Placental insufficiency

(D) An esophageal fistula

(E) Maternal malnutrition

15. Which of the following would be the best in utero test for diagnosing anencephaly or myeloschisis?

(A) Ultrasound and amniocentesis

(B) Chorionic villi sampling

(C) Measuring maternal corticosteroid levels

(D) Percutaneous umbilical blood sampling

(E) Karyotyping

16. Early viable fetuses generally have all of the following characteristics except:

(A) They usually weigh more than 500 gm.

(B) Their fingernails and toenails are well developed and lanugo hair has been replaced.

(C) They have significant amounts of body fat.

(D) If male, their testes have descended into the scrotum.

(E) Alveolar type II cells are present and secreting surfactant.

17. Nutrients and oxygen must pass through several barriers to reach the fetal blood. Which of the following represents the sequential order of these barriers during the third trimester, starting from the maternal sinusoids?

(A) Maternal sinusoids → cytotrophoblasts → chorionic mesoderm → fetal capillary endothelium

(B) Maternal sinusoids → syncytiotrophoblasts → chorionic mesoderm → fetal capillary endothelium

(C) Maternal sinusoids → syncytiotrophoblasts → fetal capillary endothelium

(D) Maternal sinusoids → cytotrophoblasts → fetal capillary endothelium

(E) Maternal sinusoids → fetal capillary endothelium

18. A patient needs a pacemaker. The cardiologist plans to run the pacemaker electrode into the right atrium via the left subclavian vein. As the cardiologist monitors placement of the catheter using angiography, the cardiologist discovers that the catheter will not enter the superior vena cava. Rather, it enters the coronary sinus and then the right atrium. How is this possible?

(A) The left supracardinal venous system did not regress during development.

(B) The patient has a left superior vena cava.

(C) The patient has a patent foramen ovale.

(D) During development, the patient's early heart tube did not loop and bend.

(E) The patient has a patent ductus arteriosus.

19. A new female patient comes to your office, and you measure her blood pressure using her right arm. It was 70 mm Hg/50 mm Hg. However, when using her left arm, you found it to be 115 mm Hg/80 mm Hg. The radial pulse was weak on the right but strong on the left. When asked, the patient said that she occasionally had difficulty swallowing. What could be a congenital basis for these observations?

(A) The patient could have a preductal coarctation of the aorta.

(B) The patient could have a postductal coarctation of the aorta.

(C) The patient could have an interrupted aortic arch.

(D) The patient could have a patent ductus arteriosus.

(E) The patient could have an anomalous origin for the right subclavian artery.

20. What forms the right subclavian artery?

(A) Aortic arch 3 and the dorsal aorta

(B) Only the seventh intersegmental artery

(C) Aortic arch 6 and the dorsal aorta

(D) Aortic arch 4, the dorsal aorta, and the seventh intersegmental artery

(E) Aortic arch 3 and the seventh intersegmental artery

Questions 21 and 22.
A newborn exhibits craniofacial anomalies, cardiac defects, immunodeficiencies, and severe hypocalcemia. Within 2 days the newborn dies. Autopsy results show thymic agenesis and an absence of parathyroid glands.

21. What is your initial diagnosis?

(A) DiGeorge syndrome

(B) Hirschsprung's disease

(C) Pierre Robin syndrome

(D) Treacher Collins syndrome

(E) First arch syndrome

22. What is one etiological basis for this syndrome?

(A) Endodermal hypoplasia in pharyngeal pouches 3 and 4

(B) A deficiency of neural crest cells in pharyngeal arches 3 and 4

(C) Congenital absence of pharyngeal clefts 3 and 4

(D) Deficiency in somitomeric mesodermal cell migration and proliferation

(E) Failed fusion between the tuberculum impar and copula

23. A 22-year-old pregnant woman revisited her obstetrician because she noticed a swelling in her right groin. She first became aware of the swelling about a month and a half into her pregnancy, but now almost 2 months later it is much larger. Examination by the physician revealed a firm swelling just to the right of the anterior abdominal wall and above the medial inguinal ligament. The swelling was located just beneath the skin, and there was a small pigmented molelike structure on the skin surface overlying the swelling. What is the most likely explanation?

(A) The woman has polymastia.

(B) The woman has polythelia.

(C) The woman has a melanoma.

(D) The woman has a hemangioma.

(E) The woman has an inguinal hernia.

24. A baby is born with an irregularly shaped red blotch on the skin overlying the right zygomatic arch. It is approximately 2 cm in diameter. If lightly pressed, it becomes temporarily blanched. What is this?

(A) Amelia

(B) Ichthyosis

(C) A capillary hemangioma

(D) An ectodermal dysplasia

(E) Piebald skin

25. In an initial examination of a newborn, you discover the presence of 2 erupted teeth on the mandible. Radiological examination showed only 1 set of underlying dental primordia. What are these teeth?

(A) Horner's teeth

(B) Supernumerary teeth

(C) Hutchinson's teeth

(D) Secondary teeth

(E) Natal teeth

26. A 6-year-old girl with a history of ear infections and chronic respiratory infections was rushed into the emergency department with acute abdominal pain symptomatic of appendicitis. However, the pain was located in the area of the left iliac fossa. An emergency appendectomy was performed, and the surgeon discovered that the appendix was on the left and all of the viscera, including the heart, were in a reversed orientation. What is this condition called?

(A) Situs inversus

(B) Dextrocardia

(C) Situs ambiguus

(D) Heterotaxia

(E) Malrotation of the gut

27. A physician informed a patient that she was pregnant, and the patient asked, "What is the expected due date for the baby?" She told the physician that her last menstrual period started on August 15. If the patient had a history of regular menstrual periods, what would be your best-estimated time of delivery?

(A) May 15

(B) May 22

(C) May 29

(D) June 15

(E) June 5

28. A pregnant woman in her third trimester telephones; she thinks that she has started labor. What sign(s) and symptom(s) would be expected if she was indeed entering labor?

(A) Painful, rhythmic uterine contractions, with each contraction occurring <10 minutes apart

(B) Dilatation of cervix

(C) Vaginal discharge of blood-stained mucus from the cervix

(D) Discharge of amniotic fluid

(E) All of the above

29. A 45-year-old female patient has pulmonary hypertension and evidence of right ventricular hypertrophy on an electrocardiogram. Further examination reveals an atrial septal defect near the upper rim of the fossa ovalis. What was the most likely cause of this defect?

(A) Excessive resorption of septum secundum

(B) Inadequate development of septum secundum

(C) Failure of atrioventricular endocardial cushion tissue to form

(D) Inadequate neural crest cell migration and proliferation

(E) Failure of ostium primum to close

30. What are the major causative factors leading to birth defects?

(A) Environmental factors

(B) Genetic factors

(C) Multifactorial inheritance

(D) Unknown factors

(E) Teratogens

31. A female patient shows signs of pregnancy, including elevated hCG levels. After consultation with the patient, you find that her last menstrual period was about 12 weeks ago. Ultrasound shows evidence of an abnormal conceptus, and chorionic villi biopsy and subsequent karyotyping show that the conceptus is triploidy. What is your diagnosis?

(A) The patient has an ectopic pregnancy.

(B) The patient has a partial molar pregnancy.

(C) The patient has a complete molar pregnancy.

(D) The patient has developed a choriocarcinoma.

(E) The patient has placenta previa.

ANSWERS

1. The answer is B.

With transposition of the great vessels, the aorta is connected to the right ventricle, and the pulmonary artery is connected to the left ventricle. In utero, this transposition does not present a problem because oxygenated blood enters the right atrium (via the umbilical vein) and because of right-to-left shunting in the foramen ovale and ductus arteriosus. Both ventricles experience a normal workload during gestation, and if there are no associated valvular defects, they develop normally. However, once the baby is delivered, venous blood from the right must be sent to the lungs to be oxygenated, returned to the left side, and then distributed to the rest of the body via the aorta. With transposition of the great vessels, there is no mechanism for exchange between the systemic and pulmonary circulatory systems, and without accompanying septal defects to permit some exchange, the condition is usually lethal, even with a patent ductus arteriosus.

2. The answer is D.

This ligament is the remnant of the ductus arteriosus, a vascular shunt between the pulmonary artery and aorta used during the embryonic and fetal period. It is derived from a section of the left sixth aortic arch. The corresponding section on the right side completely disappears during embryogenesis. After birth, the ductus arteriosus closes and becomes a ligament. The vagus nerve innervates the sixth pharyngeal arch, including the intrinsic musculature of the larynx. The embryonic heart is initially located in the cervical region, but differential growth carries the heart into the thorax, dragging a laryngeal branch of the vagus down with it. On the left, the recurrent laryngeal nerve remains hooked around the ductus arteriosus as it reaches for the larynx, but on the right side it is wrapped around the right subclavian artery (fourth aorta arch) because a part of the right sixth aortic arch disappears.

3. The answer is A.

Coarctation of the aorta is a congenital stenosis of the aorta. Its classification depends on whether the stenosis is upstream or downstream of the ductus arteriosus (preductal or postductal, respectively). With postductal coarctation, oxygenated blood going to the lower body is hampered by the stenosis so that the embryo or fetus develops a large collateral circulation in order to compensate. After birth, these individuals are usually asymptomatic. In preductal coarctation,

because the ductus arteriosus shunts oxygen-rich blood from the pulmonary artery into the aorta below the coarctation, the lower body gets the oxygen that it needs and the collateral circulation is not enhanced. But after birth, this is no longer the case. Once inflated, the pulmonary artery carries only deoxygenated blood. Since enhanced collateral circulation did not develop, the only way a significant blood supply reaches the lower body is via a patent ductus arteriosus, and it will be carrying only venous blood. Therefore, depending on the degree of preductal coarctation, the lower body may be extremely cyanotic, and this condition can lead to death. This defect can usually be repaired surgically.

4 and 5. The answers are C and B, respectively.

Initially, 2 umbilical veins run from the umbilicus to the sinus venosus of the heart. These veins pass through the developing sinusoids of the liver and carry oxygenated blood to the heart. The distal right umbilical vein degenerates early in development while a shunt called the ductus venosus develops within the liver. The ductus venosus permits much of the blood carried by the left umbilical vein to bypass the liver sinusoids and empty directly into the inferior vena cava. As the abdominal cavity and liver develop, the left umbilical vein becomes wrapped within folds of peritoneum, forming the falciform ligament. After birth, the umbilical vein and ductus venosum close off, and these vessels become ligaments easily recognized within the adult (ligamentum teres hepatis and ligamentum venosum, respectively).

6. The answer is A.

In this case, the tricuspid valve did not develop properly, and the right atrioventricular canal was obliterated. Consequently, blood did not enter the right ventricle, which became hypoplastic. In addition, all of the blood returning to the heart entered the systemic circulation via the foramen ovale; therefore, the entire workload for pumping blood was put on the left ventricle. This led to left ventricular hypertrophy. This situation is compatible with life in utero. But after birth, oxygenated blood no longer enters the right atrium, and it must now be oxygenated in the neonatal lungs. In this situation, the only means of getting blood to the lungs is by way of a patent foramen ovale and patent ductus arteriosus. Blood could also be shunted to the pulmonary side through an accompanying VSD, if present. Tricuspid atresia can be surgically corrected provided the right ventricular hypoplasia and left ventricular hypertrophy are not too severe. Otherwise, the newborn may require a heart transplant.

7. The answer is B.

The most common cause of cyanosis in newborns is tetralogy of Fallot. This condition arises because of an unequal division of the cardiac outflow tract, resulting in pulmonary artery stenosis, an aorta overriding into the right ventricle, and a VSD. Because of the pulmonary stenosis, the right ventricle hypertrophies. By the time of birth, the right ventricle usually has hypertrophied to the point that once the lungs inflate, right-to-left shunting through the VSD ensues, causing cyanosis. The right ventricular hypertrophy progresses, eventually leading to heart failure if not surgically corrected. Neural crest cells play a key role in the formation of the conotruncal septum as well as cranial facial primordia. The co-expression of conotruncal defects with cleft lip and palate suggests that neural crest morphogenesis was abnormal in this child. In fact, a large percentage of children with craniofacial anomalies have conotruncal and ventricular defects.

8. The answer is C.

The earliest hematopoiesis begins with the formation of blood islands in the yolk sac mesoderm. Soon after, hematopoiesis expands into the chorionic mesoderm and umbilical cord mesoderm. Hemocytoblasts later populate the liver, which becomes the next major hematopoietic organ, and blood cells are continually produced at this site until late in the fetal period. During the fetal period, the spleen becomes a temporary hematopoietic organ as well. Eventually, hematopoiesis shifts to the bone marrow, and bone marrow remains the major site of hematopoiesis in the newborn and adult. Vasculogenesis in the intraembryonic mesoderm is not coupled with hematopoiesis.

9. The answer is C.

In a single birth pregnancy, the trophoblast of the developing blastula forms the placenta while the inner cell mass forms the embryo. As the inner cell mass develops, the amniotic cavity forms between the inner cell mass and trophoblast. In this multiple birth, the twins shared a single placenta. Therefore, they developed from single blastula with 2 separate inner cell masses as they had separate amniotic cavities. If the twins had developed from a split zygote, 2 separate blastulae would develop, producing twins, each with its own placenta. And, if they had developed from a single inner cell mass with 2 bilaminar disks, they would have a common amniotic cavity.

10. The answer is C.

VSDs are the most common heart defect. With a VSD, both heart chambers develop normally in utero. However, after birth with the expansion of the lungs, pulmonary resistance decreases with a concomitant decrease in right ventricular pressure. Increased blood flow through the lungs increases blood return into the left atrium and ventricle, thereby increasing left ventricular pressure. With VSD, this causes a left-to-right shunting of blood through the defect. This is acyanotic. Because of the increased workload, the right ventricle begins to hypertrophy and pulmonary congestion ensues. Eventually, right ventricular pressure will exceed the systemic pressure and right-to-left shunting begins through the VSD, leading to cyanosis. If not corrected, this will lead to congestive heart failure and death. The rate at which these complications appear depends on the size of the VSD.

11. The answer is E.

Excessive amniotic fluid is called hydramnios; when extremely excessive, it is referred to as polyhydramnios. The turnover of amniotic fluid depends

on a balance between secretion and removal. Amniotic fluid usually is removed by fetal swallowing and uptake by the fetal GI tract (ultimately transported to the mother via the placenta). If the fetus is unable to swallow or if the fluid cannot pass through the GI tract for any reason, hydramnios or polyhydramnios results. Esophageal atresia usually leads to polyhydramnios because it is a form of GI obstruction. However, the elevated α-fetoprotein level suggests that this fetus may be anencephalic. Without a functional brain, the fetus cannot generate swallowing motions, thereby leading to polyhydramnios. α-Fetoprotein is secreted primarily by the liver but is produced in much smaller amounts by other cells; thus, it is normally found at low levels within the amniotic fluid. However, in cases of NTDs, gastroschisis, and exstrophy of the bladder, large amounts of α-fetoprotein are released into the amniotic fluid.

12. The answer is B.

If the mother was Rh-negative and her first child was Rh-positive, there is a good chance that the mother was immunized with Rh protein because of blood leakage at the maternal sinusoid-villi interface. At birth, even more mixing of blood occurs. Consequently, the mother develops antibodies against the Rh factor, and these antibodies cross the placental barrier. In a pregnancy carrying a second Rh-positive fetus, the Rh antibody titers will be higher. Since these antibodies cross the placenta and bind the fetal RBCs, the fetal RBCs lyse, resulting in hemolytic disease (erythroblastosis fetalis). If severe enough, this can threaten the life of the fetus if not treated. The baby survived in this case, but the lysis of fetal RBCs led to an enlargement of the liver and spleen. These organs continued serving as hematopoietic organs to replace the lysed RBCs. The lysed RBCs released large amounts of bilirubin that initially were cleared by the mother's liver. After delivery, however, jaundice rapidly appeared in the newborn because the mother's liver was no longer clearing the bilirubin. Rh immunoglobulin therapy, particularly after the birth of each Rh-positive child, usually prevents the development of serious forms of the disease.

13. The answer is B.

Measuring the crown-rump length using ultrasonic imaging can be a very accurate means of determining gestational age (usually within 1 or 2 days). When combined with other measurements, such as biparietal head diameter, it can be even more accurate.

14. The answer is D.

Cigarette smoking, multiple births, placental insufficiency, and malnutrition, not an esophageal fistula, can increase the risk of having a low-birth-weight baby. Low-birth-weight infants have a higher risk of infant mortality.

15. The answer is A.

Anencephaly and myeloschisis, both NTDs, dramatically increase the levels of α-fetoprotein in amniotic fluid. Ultrasound methods alone may enable visualization of these defects, but amniocentesis and α-fetoprotein measurements would support the diagnosis.

16. The answer is D.

All these characteristics are found in viable fetuses with the exception of testicular descent. In males, the testes do not descend until late in the fetal period and, in some cases, may not be completed within the first year of birth in normal infants. Testicular descent is not a characteristic associated with fetal viability.

17. The answer is C.

Nutrients and oxygen must cross over several layers of tissue before reaching the fetal bloodstream during the embryonic period and early fetal period. But because of a loss of some of the cytotrophoblasts and intervening chorionic mesoderm by the third trimester, the placental-fetal barrier is reduced to only a thin layer of syncytiotrophoblasts and fetal capillary endothelial cells.

18. The answer is B.

Early in the development of the venous system, blood from the head and upper part of the body empties into the sinus venosus by way of the anterior and common cardinal veins and the sinus horns. An anastomosis develops between the right and left anterior cardinal veins so that the venous drainage from the upper left side of the body enters the right anterior and common cardinal veins (future superior vena cava). Once established, the left cardinal system and left sinus horn degenerate, and all that remains is a small segment forming the coronary sinus and oblique vein. If the anastomosis fails to form, the left anterior and common cardinal veins are retained and form a left superior vena cava, which serves to return venous blood from the left upper part of the body to the right atrium by way of the coronary sinus. Therefore, this patient has either a left superior vena cava or a double superior vena cava.

19. The answer is E.

In anomalous origin of the right subclavian artery, the right subclavian artery originates on the left side of the body and downstream of the origin for the left subclavian artery. To reach the right upper limb, the right subclavian artery usually runs posterior to the esophagus. This can compress the artery, reducing blood flow to the right upper limb. Likewise, compression of the esophagus between the aortic arch and anomalous right subclavian artery may cause dysphagia (difficulty swallowing). The decrease in blood pressure also could occur in this situation if there was a coarctation between the origin of the left subclavian artery and anomalous origin of the right subclavian artery.

20. The answer is D.

The right subclavian artery is formed from several different arterial segments. These include the right fourth aortic arch, the right seventh intersegmental artery, and the intervening segment of the right dorsal aorta. In contrast, the left subclavian artery is derived only from the seventh intersegmental artery.

21 and 22. The answers are A and B, respectively.

DiGeorge syndrome is characterized by the partial or complete agenesis of the parathyroid glands and thymus gland. It is often accompanied by craniofacial defects (e.g., microagnathia, hypertelorism, ear anomalies) and cardiovascular defects. It can occur as a consequence of a partial deletion of chromosome 22 or maternal alcohol consumption during the embryonic period. The spectrum of defects is thought to be due to abnormal morphogenesis of neural crest cells, particularly those entering the pharyngeal arches. Neural crest cell–derived mesenchyme in pharyngeal arches 3 and 4 is essential for the normal development of the thymus and parathyroid glands (calcitonin-producing cells are neural crest–derived). Neural crest cells in pharyngeal arches 3, 4, and 6 are also involved in cardiac septation. Agenesis of the thymus glands and parathyroid glands leads to serious immunodeficiencies and hypocalcemia, respectively. The prognosis is poor.

23. The answer is A.

The woman has an accessory breast on the right side (polymastia). The accessory mammary gland was located along the milkline in the inguinal region. In response to the hormones associated with pregnancy, the accessory mammary tissue began to proliferate and respond to the hormones in the same manner as the pectoral mammary glands. The swollen accessory mammary tissue became painful and tender during pregnancy. After pregnancy, it will shrink in size and return to its previous state. After pregnancy, she can opt to have it surgically removed.

24. The answer is C.

Capillary hemangioma (nevus vascularis) of the skin is relatively common and results from an abnormal vasculogenesis and angiogenesis of the skin capillaries. The red coloration is due to a high density of capillaries and the fact that oxygen levels are higher in this area because of the increased density of blood vessels. Capillary hemangiomas range from physically harmless ones, as in the case of the skin (birthmark), to those that continue to grow and form vascular tangles with clinical consequences (e.g., in the brain, these tangles can restrict blood flow, leading to central nervous system dysfunction including epileptic seizures).

25. The answer is E.

The presence of natal teeth is most often due to a premature eruption of the primary teeth rather than the supernumerary teeth. Natal teeth occur in about 1/2,000 births and can lead to complications, particularly concerning maternal comfort during breast-feeding. Natal teeth usually develop in the region normally occupied by the mandibular incisors. If natal teeth are supernumerary, they are usually removed, because they may interfere with the normal development of the underlying primary teeth.

26. The answer is A.

With situs inversus, orientation of both the heart and the viscera is reversed. While there are no major physiological consequences of situs inversus, there is a propensity for these individuals to develop ear and respiratory infections and have reduced fertility. Reverse orientation of the heart is called dextrocardia and develops as a consequence of abnormal cardiac looping. Rarely does dextrocardia occur without a concomitant reversal of the other organs. However, when this does occur, it is called heterotaxia or situs ambiguus and often leads to the development of congenital anomalies in the venous system to the heart.

27. The answer is B.

Since the patient has fairly regular menstrual cycles and provided a reliable date for the onset of her last menstrual period, you can calculate the estimated delivery date by subtracting 3 months from the starting date of the last menstrual period and then adding 1 year plus 7 days (August 15, 2000 minus 3 months is May 15, 2000, and add 1 year and 7 days, which is May 22, 2001). This method can be accurate if the patient remembers the onset date of her last menstrual period and is not confusing it with possible implantation bleeding. As the pregnancy progresses, you can get a closer estimate of gestational age by performing ultrasonic imaging and obtaining length measurements.

28. The answer is E.

All these are symptoms of labor.

29. The answer is B.

During atrial septation, 2 muscular septa form, septum primum and septum secundum. As ostium primum is closed by atrioventricular cushion tissue, ostium secundum develops in the upper part of septum primum. Meanwhile, septum secundum begins growing and overlaps ostium secundum but never completely spans the atrium, thereby leaving an opening called the foramen ovale. Blood passes from the right atrium to the left atrium through the foramen ovale but not in the reverse direction, because septum primum acts as a 1-way valve. Given the available choices, the defect was most likely caused by inadequate development of septum secundum since the defect was near the upper rim of the fossa ovalis. However, excessive resorption of septum primum, leading to the formation of an enlarged ostium secundum, could also generate a similar defect. Failure of ostium primum to close was unlikely since the defect was not near the atrioventricular valves. In atrial septal defects, left-to-right shunting of blood occurs after birth when the systemic pressure exceeds the pulmonary pressure. Eventually, this leads to right ventricular hypertrophy and pulmonary hypertension. Atrial septal defects are fairly well tolerated during childhood, but by adulthood, symptoms begin to appear at an age that depends in part on the size of the defect. Atrial septal defects are more prevalent in females than males (2:1).

30. **The answer is D.**

Between 50% and 60% of congenital defects are of unknown etiology. Fifteen percent are caused by genetic factors, with the likelihood that more will be discovered. Environmental factors are thought to cause about 10% of congenital defects while a combination of environmental and genetic factors (multifactorial) is thought to contribute to about 20%–25% of congenital defects.

31. **The answer is B.**

Partial molar pregnancies result from a triploidy condition. These zygotes develop trophoblastic tissue and an inner cell mass. The inner cell mass goes on to various degrees of development, but triploidy embryos are usually aborted very early. Triploidy is thought to occur as a consequence of dispermic fertilization of a single ovum and fusion of the 3 pronuclei. Complete moles do not develop an inner cell mass and, if not fully removed, eventually form metastatic choriocarcinomas. Complete moles are thought to occur as a consequence of either dispermy with a concomitant loss of the maternal pronuclei or male pronucleus duplication followed by male pronuclear fusion within the oocyte and then loss of the maternal pronuclei. Because both types of molar pregnancies generate trophoblastic tissue, the patient exhibits symptoms of pregnancy.

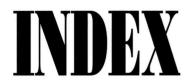

INDEX

Fetal alcohol syndrome, 115, 67, 73, 76, 108, 109
Fetal period, 96–97
    α-Fetoprotein, neural tube defect-related increase in, 111, 114
Fetus, viability assessment of, 97, 111, 114
Fingerprints, 95
First arch syndrome, 53, 61
Fistulas
    between rectum, bladder, and vagina, 45
    omphalomesenteric/umbilical, 36, 37
    rectoprostatic, 37
    rectourethral, 37
    rectouterine, 37
    rectovaginal, 37
    tracheoesophageal, 24, 25
    urachal, 40, 41
Folic acid deficiency, 26, 29
Follicles, ovarian
    atretic, 5,
    development of, 4, 5, 7
    estrogen secretion by, 7
    as graafian follicles, 4, 5
    primordial, 45
Follicle-stimulating hormone, 28, 30
    during menstrual cycle, 6, 7
    oocyte-stimulating activity of, 5
Fontanelles, 51
Foramen cecum, 56, 57, 116
Foramen of Monro, 63, 66, 67
Foramen ovale, 82, 83
    closure of, 104, 105
    patent, 82, 83, 85
Forebrain (prosencephalon), 62, 63, 66–67
Foregut
    derivatives of, 33, 35
    development of, 25, 32–33
    formation of, 22, 23
Fornix commissure, 66, 67
Friedreich's syndrome/ataxia, 65, 73, 76

G

Gallbladder, 33, 35
Gametes. See also Oocytes; Spermatozoa
    possible types of, 3
Gametogenesis
    female, 4–5
    male, 8–9
Gartner's cyst, 45
Gastrointestinal tract, development of
    of duodenum and accessory glands, 34–35
    of foregut and stomach, 32–33
    of midgut and foregut, 36–37
Gastrosplenic ligament, 68, 74
Gastroschisis, 23
    differentiated from omphacele, 37
Gastrulation, 16–17
    neural plate formation during, 18, 19
Gaucher's disease, 107
Gene therapy, 107

Genetic factors, in congenital anomalies, 108, 109
Genitalia. See also Gonads; Reproductive system
    female, 44, 45
    male, 42
Germ cells, primordial
    male, 5, 8, 9, 42
    origin of, 4
Germ cells, primordial, 26, 29
    female, 4, 5, 44, 45
Germ layers, developmental sequence of, 27, 30
Gestational age, estimation of, 96, 111, 114
Glaucoma, congenital, 59
Glioblasts, 62, 63
Glucagon-secreting cells, 35
Glucocorticoids, as respiratory distress syndrome
    prophylaxis, 25
Glycogen, placental synthesis of, 101
Gonadal cancer, pseudohermaphroditism-related, 47
Gonadal ridges, 44, 45
Gonadotropin-releasing hormone, during menstrual cycle, 7
Gonadotropins, ovulation-inducing activity of, 5
Gonadotropin therapy, use in in vitro fertilization, 27, 29
Gonads
    indifferent, 43
    male, differentiation of, 70, 74
    mesenteries of, 46, 47
Graafian follicles, 4, 5
Granulocytes, 92, 93
Granulosa cells, 5
Greater omentum, 32, 33
Growth, fetal, 96, 97
Growth impairment. See also Intrauterine
    growth restriction (IUGR)
        maternal alcohol use-related, 67
Gubernaculum, 46, 47
Gut, early folding and formation of, 22–23

H

Hair, 94, 95
    congenital absence of, 95
    lanugo, 95
Head, during fetal period, 96, 97
Head and neck, development of
    axial skeleton, 50–51
    craniofacial anomalies in, 51, 52–53, 55, 57, 59, 61, 65, 67
    face, 52–53
    musculature, 50–51
    pharyngeal arches, pouches, and grooves, 52–53
    pituitary gland, 56–57
    thyroid gland, 56–57
    tongue, 56–57
Heart
    atrial septation, 82–83
    early phase, 80–81
    outflow septation in, 84, 85
    ventricular septation in, 84, 85
Heart defects, 81. See also specific heart defects
    maternal alcohol use-related, 67

Middle ear, development of, 60, 61
Midgut
    derivatives of, 35
    development of, 32, 33, 36, 37
    physiological umbilical herniation of, 37
    rotation of, 36, 37
Mirror-image reversal, of asymmetrical organs, 81
Mitosis, 2, 3
Monocytes, 92, 93
Monosomy, 109
Monro, interventricular foramen of, 63, 66, 67
    closure of, 85
Morula, 10, 11, 29
    as chimera source, 12, 13
    compaction of, 11
    use in *in vitro* fertilization, 13
Mothers, surrogate, 13, 27, 29
Mouth, primordial, 33
Müllerian-inhibiting substance, 42, 43, 45
    in pseudohermaphroditism, 47
Multiple births, 102–103
    as low-birth-weight risk factor, 111, 114
Musculature
    development of, 50–51
    laryngeal, 87
    ocular, 59
    skeletal, 49
Mutations, as congenital anomalies cause, 108, 109
Myelencephalon, 62, 63, 64, 65
Myeloschisis (rachischisis), 18, 19
    in utero for, 111, 114
Myocardium, 80, 81, 82
Myocytes, 48, 49
Myometrium, uterine, 6, 7
    post-delivery contraction of, 105
Myotome cells, in prune-belly syndrome, 28, 30
Myotomes, 20, 21

N

Nasal cavity, 52, 53
Nasal processes, lateral and medial, 52, 53
Nasal septum, 52, 53
Nasolacrimal groove, 52, 53
Neck, development of. *See* Head and neck, development of
Nervous system, development of, 18–19
    adrenal gland, 68, 69
    cranial nerves, 68, 69
    early, 62–63
    forebrain, 66–67
    hindbrain, 64–65
    midbrain, 66–67
    peripheral nervous system, 66–67, 68, 69
    spinal cord, 62–63
Neural crest, 18, 19
Neural crest cells, 69
    abnormal morphogenesis of, 26, 28
    cardiac, 84, 85
    pharyngeal arch deficiency in, 112, 115
Neural crest-derived cell tumors, 18

Neural elements, 62, 63
Neural plate, 18, 19
Neural tube, 69
    brain segment of, 64–65
    early, 62, 63
    neuroepithelial cells of, 72–73, 76
    spinal cord segment of, 62–63
Neural tube defects, 18, 19, 63
    α-fetoprotein increase in, 111, 114
    folic acid deficiency-related, 26, 29
Neuroblasts, 63, 67
    of the basal plates, 73, 76
Neurocranium, 50, 51
Neurocristopathies, 18, 19
Neuroepithelial cells, 62, 63, 72–73, 76
Neurofibromatosis (von Recklinghausen's disease), 18
Neurulation, 18, 19
    abnormal, 19
Nipples, 94, 95
    supernumerary, 95
Notochord, 16, 17
Nuclei, neuronal, 65
Nutrients
    fetal blood vessel transport of, 105
    placental transport of, 100, 101, 111, 115
Nutritional deficiencies, as congenital anomalies cause, 108, 109

O

Oblique vein, 91
Odontoblasts, 94, 95
Offspring, sex determination of, 13
Olfactory bulb, 66, 67
Oligodendroglia, 62, 63
Oligohydramnios, 101
    as limb defect cause, 49
    renal agenesis-related, 39
Omental bursa, 33
Omphacele, 36, 37, 70, 74
    differentiated from gastroschisis, 37
Oocytes. *See also* Ovum
    degeneration of, 45
    development of. *See* Oogenesis
    penetration of, 10, 11
    secondary meiotic division of, 11
Oogenesis, 4, 5
    in 2-chromosome organisms, 4, 5
Oogonia
    formation of, 4, 44, 45
    proliferation and differentiation of, 5, 45
Optic chiasma, 66, 67
Optic cup, 58, 59
Optic stalk, 67
Optic vesicles, 58, 59, 63, 67
    weak adhesion within, 72, 75
Organ of Corti, 61
Organogenesis, period of, 17
Organs, asymmetrical, mirror-image reversal of, 81

Skull
    anomalies of, 51
    development of, 50–51
Small intestine, 33
Smoking
    as intrauterine growth retardation cause, 109
    as low-birth-weight cause, 111, 114
Smooth muscle, 33
Somatopleure, 20, 21
Somatostatin-secreting cells, 35
Somites, 20, 21
    cranial skeletal, 50, 51
    paraxial, as fetal age indicators, 97
Somitomeres, 20, 21
    cranial skeletal, 50, 51
Spermatic cord, 46, 47
Spermatids, 8, 9
Spermatocytes
    primary, 8, 9
    secondary, 8, 9
Spermatogenesis, 8, 9
Spermatogonia, 8, 9
Spermatozoa, 8, 9
    during fertilization, 10, 11
    lifespan of, 26, 28
    maturation (capacitation) of, 9
        artificial, 27, 29
    zona pellucida binding by, 10, 11
        blockage of, 26, 29
    zona pellucida penetration by, 10, 11
Sperm count, 9
Spina bifida occulta, 18, 19
Spinal cord, development and organization of, 62–63
Spinal cord defects, 18, 19, 63
Spinal nerves, 20, 49, 68, 69
Splanchnic mesoderm
    intraembryoinic, 20, 21
    precardiac, 81
Splanchnopleure, 20, 21
Spleen
    development of, 92, 93
    as hematopoietic organ, 92, 93
Stapedial artery, 87
Stapes, 71, 75
Stem cells, 92, 93
    embryonic, 12, 13
    epidermal, 95
    hematopoietic, 92, 93
    male reproductive, 26, 29
Sterility
    definition of, 13
    male, 9
Sternocleidomastoid muscle, 54, 55
Stomach, 32, 33
Stomodeum, 52, 53
Stratum germinativum, 95
Stratum granulosa, 4, 5
Subarachnoid space, 63
Subclavian arteries
    left, 86

Subclavian arteries (cont.)
    right, 113
        anomalous, 88, 89, 111–112, 115
        formation of, 86, 112, 115
Superior intercostal artery, 87
Superior vena cava, 80, 81, 91
    anomalies of, 90, 91
    left, 111, 115
Supradrenal (adrenal) gland, 68, 69
Surgery, intrauterine corrective, 107
Surrogate mothers, 13, 27, 29
Sweat glands, 94, 95
    congenital absence of, 95
Sylvius, aqueduct of, 62, 63, 66, 67
    blockage of, 73, 76
Sympathetic ganglia, 68, 69
Sympathetic nervous system, 68, 69
Synapsis, in meiotic cells, 28, 30
Syncytial knots, 98, 99
Syncytiotrophoblasts, 10, 11, 14, 98, 99, 100, 111, 115
Syndactyly, 48, 71, 75
Syphilis, placental transmission of, 100, 101

T

Taste buds, 57
Tectorial membrane, 60, 61
Teeth
    development of, 94, 95
    natal, 95, 112, 115
Tegmentum of the mesencephalon, 67
Telencephalon, 62, 63, 66, 67
Telophase, of mitosis and meiosis, 2, 3
Teratogens, 108, 109
    as limb defect cause, 49
    placental transmission of, 100, 101
Teratology, 109
Teratoma, sacrococcygeal, 17, 28, 30
Testes
    cryptorchid, 47, 71, 75
    descent of, 46, 47, 111, 114
    development of, 42, 43
    prepubescent, 8, 9
Testicular feminization syndrome, 47
Testis-determining factor, 43, 70, 74
Testosterone, Leydig cell production of, 43
Tetralogy of Fallot, 84, 85, 110, 114
Thalamus, 62
Thalidomide, teratogenicity of, 49
Thoracopagus, 102, 103
Thymocytes, 93
Thymus, 54, 55
    development of, 92, 93
    as hematopoietic organ, 92, 93
Thyroglossal cysts, 56, 57, 72, 76
Thyroglossal duct, 56, 57
Thyroid gland, 56, 57
Thyroxine, 57
Tibial defects, partial, 49
Tissue culture, use in in vitro fertilization, 27, 29